Multiple Sclerosis

T0201373

Multiple Sclerosis

A Practical Manual for Hospital and Outpatient Care

Carlos A. Pérez
The University of Texas Health Science Center at Houston

Andrew Smith
University of Minnesota

Flavia Nelson
University of Minnesota

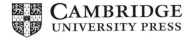

CAMBRIDGE
UNIVERSITY PRESS

CAMBRIDGE
UNIVERSITY PRESS

University Printing House, Cambridge CB2 8BS, United Kingdom

One Liberty Plaza, 20th Floor, New York, NY 10006, USA

477 Williamstown Road, Port Melbourne, VIC 3207, Australia

314–321, 3rd Floor, Plot 3, Splendor Forum, Jasola District Centre,
New Delhi – 110025, India

79 Anson Road, #06–04/06, Singapore 079906

Cambridge University Press is part of the University of Cambridge.

It furthers the University's mission by disseminating knowledge in the pursuit of
education, learning, and research at the highest international levels of excellence.

www.cambridge.org
Information on this title: www.cambridge.org/9781108820752
DOI: 10.1017/9781108907484

First published 2021

Printed in the United Kingdom by TJ Books Limited, Padstow Cornwall

A catalogue record for this publication is available from the British Library.

ISBN 978-1-108-82075-2 Paperback

....

Contents

Preface

Multiple sclerosis (MS) is the most prevalent nontraumatic, disabling neurologic condition among young adults worldwide. The diagnosis and management of MS are complicated, especially in the setting of a recent significant increase in the number of Food and Drug Administration–approved therapies, and access to neurologic care, specifically to MS centers, is limited. The goal of this handbook is to present an updated and practical approach to the accurate diagnosis and effective management of MS, for both healthcare professionals and trainees, in hopes of improving patient outcomes. The material presented in this text is meant to be an easily accessible resource for reference in both hospital and outpatient practice settings.

The first chapter addresses the unique aspects of acute MS exacerbations, with a focus on timely recognition and management to facilitate urgent decision-making in the emergency room. In addition to MS, related neuroimmunologic conditions including transverse myelitis and optic neuritis are discussed. The following chapters discuss various aspects of MS ranging from clinical features and diagnosis to long-term management and treatment goals. Because MS usually affects women during their childbearing years, a dedicated chapter on pregnancy and reproductive issues is presented. Lastly, since MS is increasingly being recognized in patients younger than 18 years, the unique aspects of pediatric-onset MS are discussed in a separate chapter.

It is important to recognize that there is no consensus on the best approach to manage patients with MS. Ongoing multicenter clinical trials are in the process of comparing outcomes using escalation versus high-efficacy drugs as first-line agents, as well as autologous hematopoietic stem cell transplant versus high-efficacy drugs, for the management of aggressive MS. Despite the continuous evolution of the treatment paradigms, the primary goal of patient care – timely recognition and treatment to decrease the risk of permanent disability – remains unchanged. The information presented in this volume is based on both current evidence where it exists, as well as our best interpretation of effective management practices where conclusive data are currently lacking. We hope this handbook will serve as a framework for providing practical insights into the management of our patients with this challenging disease.

Chapter 1

Autoimmune CNS Emergencies

Andrew Smith, MD

Introduction

The primary role of the neurologist in the emergency department (ED) when confronted with a potential exacerbation of a neuroimmunologic condition is first, to rule out potential "mimics," and second, to treat acute episodes of true neurologic dysfunction.

- True neuroimmunologic emergencies are relatively rare ED presentations.
- Most patients with a known neuroimmunologic condition such as multiple sclerosis (MS) present to the ED with a non-neurologic issue or a "pseudorelapse."[1]

MS Relapses

A relapse (also referred to as an exacerbation, flare, or attack) is defined as "new or acutely worsening neurological symptoms lasting 24–48 hours and separated by at least 30 days from the onset of the last relapse."[1,2] These symptoms must be constant (not off and on) and accompanied by an objective change in neurologic exam, with no other explanation (such as fever, infection exhaustion, or dehydration).

Relapse vs. Pseudorelapse
Relapse

- New or worsening *constant* symptoms lasting at least 24–48 hours.
- Usually associated with inflammation and demyelination in the central nervous system (CNS) on magnetic resonance imaging (MRI; enhancing the lesion in a post-gadolinium T1-weighted image).
- Post-contrast imaging must be acquired 5 minutes after gadolinium is administered.
- Separated from the last exacerbation by at least 30 days.

Pseudorelapse

- Temporary flare-up of *old* symptom(s) lasting *less than 24 hours*, typically described as "off-and-on" symptoms.
- Symptoms are not associated with CNS inflammation (no enhancement on MRI).
- Possible triggers: increased core body temperature due to infection, exposure to heat and humidity, overexertion, bladder or bowel fullness, and/or stress.
- Symptoms usually return to baseline when the trigger is eliminated, though it may take days in the case of infection or physical exhaustion.

Assessment of a Relapse

Determining whether a person is having a true relapse can be challenging, but is important before initiating steroid treatment. Evaluation for underlying causes is imperative:

- Screen for underlining infections with a urinary albumin to urinary creatinine ratio (UAUC), complete blood count (CBC), and possibly chest x-ray. Frequently, pseudorelapses are related to an underlying infection, most commonly a urinary tract infection (UTI) or upper respiratory infection (URI). It is important to note that patients with MS often do not have the normal signs and symptoms of a UTI, and a urine test must be performed despite a lack of presenting classic UTI symptoms.
- If presenting symptoms are acute versus subacute, consider evaluation for a vascular cause.
- Symptoms that rarely represent an MS relapse include low back pain, chest pain, altered mental status, aphasia, and seizures; thus, other causes should be considered in the differential diagnosis and further evaluation is necessary.

Treatment

- Treat any identified underlying causes.
- Avoid steroids if it is not a clear MS relapse.
- Have the patient notify and follow up with the treating neurologist as soon as possible.

Differential Diagnosis

The differential diagnosis is discussed in more detail in **Chapter 5**.

- There are multiple manifestations of autoimmune CNS conditions among patients who present to the ED.
- An important step in determining the correct etiology is establishing the onset and chronology of symptom evolution.

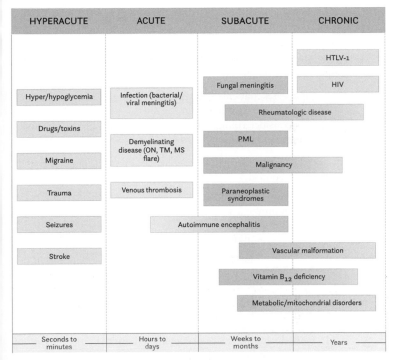

Figure 1.1 Common diagnoses according to the time course of symptom onset.

- A characteristic feature of acute demyelinating disease is gradual worsening of symptoms over the course of *hours to days*. A timeline of common alternative diagnoses based on chronological progression of symptom severity is shown in Figure 1.1.

  - If the patient's symptoms are of maximal severity at onset (within seconds to minutes), it is critical to rule out a vascular cause (i.e., stroke).
  - Patients who experience a slow and gradual onset of symptoms are less likely to present to the ED. However, it is important to keep in mind that an acute event, such as a fall, may increase patients' awareness of their slowly progressing symptoms, thereby prompting an ED visit for an unrelated reason.

- Clinicians should also consider whether the patient has any associated non-neurologic symptoms.

  - One of the most common reasons for patients to present to the ED is recrudescence of previous symptoms (**Uhthoff's phenomenon**) in the setting of a febrile illness.

    - In these cases, patients will typically return to their neurologic baseline after recovering from the illness.
    - Always consider ruling out a UTI, even if the patient does not complain of dysuria, hematuria, or frequency.

  - Always consider meningitis or encephalitis as possible diagnoses in the right clinical context.

    - Chronic immunomodulation/suppression in patients with neuroimmunologic conditions, such as MS, can increase their risk of serious infections.
    - Patients may not always present with the classic symptoms for these conditions, such as fever, headache, encephalopathy, or neck stiffness.
    - Uncommon and opportunistic infections should always be ruled out.
    - Cerebrospinal fluid (CSF) studies should always be performed in the right clinical context.
    - In individuals with space-occupying lesions, the possibility of an abscess should be considered.

  - Other symptoms that should significantly broaden the differential diagnosis include unintentional weight loss, rashes, swollen joints, and symptoms suggestive of multi-organ system involvement, which would warrant a more aggressive diagnostic workup when present.

- Once possible alternative diagnoses have been ruled out, the next step is to initiate treatment for the confirmed acute relapse.

Treatment of an Acute Relapse

- Not every acute demyelinating relapse requires acute treatment with corticosteroids.
- Typically, steroids are reserved for patients with symptoms that are severe enough to affect their ability to work or function at home.
- In MS patients with severe relapses and significant acute functional disability, clinical trials have demonstrated a benefit of treatment with high-dose intravenous (IV) corticosteroids.[2,3]

- "High" doses of steroids range from 1,000 to 2,000 mg over 3–5 days.[4–9]

  - The most common regimen is 1,000 mg of IV methylprednisolone (IVMP) for 3 days for an average mild relapse (or for 5–7 days with moderate to severe presentations).
  - An alternative dosing regimen consists of a 3- to 5-day course of 1,250 mg of oral prednisone.[9]
  - However, the highest widely available dosing formulation of prednisone is 50 mg tablets (25 pills per day).
  - The first high-dose steroid treatment must be under medical supervision, since steroids can cause a wide range of mostly mild, but potentially severe, physical and psychiatric side effects (Table 1.1).
  - If a patient tolerates the first dose of IVMP without complications and inpatient physical therapy is not indicated, oral steroids may be used to complete the course.

- With or without steroid treatment, patients generally begin to recover days to weeks after reaching peak disability, though steroids typically improve the rate of recovery.
- If the patient fails to respond to the initial steroid treatment and continues to worsen, a longer course of steroids may be considered.
- If the patient's relapse is severe and not responding to IVMP after 3–5 days, plasma exchange should be considered (typically divided into five separate treatments).[10,11]

  - There is little evidence to support treatment with adrenocorticotropic hormone (ACTH) or intravenous immunoglobulin (IVIG) when patients do not respond to steroids,[12,13] unless there is an allergy to them.
  - Because some patients may report a subjective worsening of symptoms following high-dose steroid treatment, any suspected lack of response should be confirmed with objective findings on neurologic exam.

- Aside from treating an MS relapse with corticosteroids, providers may have to treat commonly associated symptoms when present.

  - A review of all possible symptoms is beyond the scope of this chapter (see Chapter 2), but some examples include:

    - Bothersome paresthesias, which can be treated with gabapentin or tricyclic antidepressants (TCAs).
    - Trigeminal neuralgia, which is commonly treated with carbamazepine, gabapentin, or duloxetine.

Table 1.1 Side effects of corticosteroids

Common side effects
• Euphoria
• Insomnia
• Dysphoria
• Anxiety
• Depression
• Increased appetite
• Metallic taste
• Lower-extremity edema
• Headache
• Myalgia
• Easy bruising
• Acne
• Gastrointestinal distress/heartburn
• Flushing
• Palpitations
Uncommon side effects
• Anaphylaxis
• Cataract formation
• Mania
• Osteoporosis
• Osteonecrosis/aseptic necrosis
• Psychosis
Worsening comorbidities
• Diabetes mellitus
• Hypertension
• Mood disorders
• Peptic ulcer disease

- Diplopia and ophthalmoplegias, which may be conservatively treated with the use of an eye patch.
- Weakness and gait imbalance, which may require intensive physical therapy depending on severity.

Common ED Presentations of Neuroimmunologic Conditions

Optic Neuritis

- Optic neuritis is a common acute presentation in the ED. It may occur as a manifestation of MS or as an isolated event.
- Symptoms usually progress over the course of hours to days.[15]
- The cardinal symptom of optic neuritis is decreased visual acuity and pain with eye movement.

    . Complete vision loss is uncommon, occurring in fewer than 3% of cases.

- Classic signs of optic neuritis include:

    . Afferent pupillary defect.
    . Decreased visual acuity.
    . Decreased red color saturation (in approximately 85% of patients).
    . Papillitis (in about one-third of patients).

- At some point in the course of their disease, about half of MS patients will develop optic neuritis.

    . Optic neuritis (typically unilateral) may be the initial presenting symptom in about 15–20% of patients with MS.

- Bilateral optic neuritis is more common in neuromyelitis optica spectrum disorder (NMOSD) and in myelin oligodendrocyte glycoprotein (MOG) antibody disease compared to multiple sclerosis.
- In the acute setting, the same practice guidelines for treatment of acute relapses (see "Treatment of an Acute Relapse" section) are followed.
- Generally, patients notice improvement in their vision within 3 weeks from onset, when untreated.
- After an initial attack of optic neuritis, about 38% of patients will develop MS at 10 years.

    . The risk is even higher (50–60%) in those with an abnormal brain MRI (three or more typical MS lesions) at presentation.

- If the patient does not present with the typical features of optic neuritis, further workup should be performed.

    . Particular consideration should be given to vascular processes such as amaurosis fugax or temporal arteritis if the symptoms develop suddenly and the pain is not of typical character.
    . The differential diagnoses for optic neuritis are broad. Table 1.2 lists the most common causes, but this list is not an all-inclusive.

Table 1.2 Common causes of inflammatory optic neuritis

Disease	Characteristics
Multiple sclerosis[16]	• Optic neuritis, intranuclear ophthalmoplegia (INO), transverse myelitis, and cerebellar symptoms. • MRI: periventricular, cortical–juxtacortical, spinal, and infratentorial lesions. • Separation of lesions in time and space. • CSF oligoclonal bands commonly present.
Neuromyelitis optica spectrum disorder (NMOSD)[17]	• Optic neuritis and/or longitudinally extensive transverse myelitis. • Recovery may be poor. • Area postrema syndrome can also occur. • Positive anti-NMO (AQP4) antibody (diagnostic).
Acute disseminated encephalomyelitis (ADEM)	• More common in children and young adults. • Typically follows a respiratory or gastrointestinal infection. • MRI: multiple large, confluent and poorly delineated lesions. • Encephalopathy is required for diagnosis. • Recovery is typically favorable, and recurrence is rare.
Non-arteritic ischemic optic neuropathy (NAION)[18,19]	• Acute painless vision loss with poor recovery. • Swelling of the optic nerve. • Altitudinal visual field defect.
Arteritic ischemic optic neuropathy (AION)[20]	• Older adults with giant cell arteritis. • Polymyalgia rheumatica symptoms. • Headache, temporal artery tenderness. • Elevated C-reactive protein (CRP) and erythrocyte sedimentation rate (ESR).
Neurosarcoidosis[18]	• Can be bilateral up to 64% of the time. • Other cranial neuropathies, pulmonary involvement, neuroendocrine dysfunction, and transverse myelitis may also occur. • Perivascular granulomatous inflammation. • Angiotensin-converting enzyme (ACE) positive (usually but not required for diagnosis).
Granulomatosis with polyangiitis (Wegener's granulomatosis)[23]	• Sinus involvement that can spread to cause orbital disease. • Kidney and lung disease. • Anti-neutrophil cytoplasmic antibodies (ANCA) positive.

Table 1.2 (cont.)

Disease	Characteristics
Behçet syndrome[24]	• Oral and genital ulcers. • Can also cause uveitis and meningitis. • Transverse myelitis. • Common in patients of Mediterranean and Asian descent.
Inflammatory bowel disease[25]	• History of Crohn's disease or ulcerative colitis. • Increased risk of optic neuritis.
Susac's syndrome[26]	• Encephalopathy. • Hearing loss. • Branch retinal artery occlusion.
Systemic lupus erythematosus (SLE)[27]	• Rash, transverse myelitis, and neuropsychiatric symptoms. • Anti-double-stranded DNA (anti-dsDNA) and anti-Smith antibodies may be present. • Multi-organ system involvement.
Infectious/parainfectious[28,29]	• Meningitis or encephalitis. • Neuroretinitis. • Recent infection.
Toxic exposures[30]	• Use of tumor necrosis factor alpha (TFN-α), bevacizumab, erectile dysfunction treatments, methanol, or antituberculous medication.
Nutritional deficiencies[31,32]	• Deficiency of vitamin B_1 (thiamine), vitamin B_9 (folic acid) and B_{12} (cobalamin). • Ethanol abuse or malnutrition.
Leber hereditary optic neuropathy (LHON)[33]	• Common in younger men. • Subacute to chronic onset. • Painless bilateral vision loss.

Acute Transverse Myelitis

- The incidence of acute transverse myelitis is estimated to be as high as 3.1 per 100,000 person-years.[34]
- Transverse myelitis affects women more commonly than men.
- The symptoms largely depend on the location of the inflammatory lesion.
  - Patients may present with a combination of sensory, pyramidal, and autonomic symptoms below the level of the lesion.
  - Symptoms will typically evolve over a few days.
  - The transverse myelitis can be complete but is more commonly partial.

Table 1.3 Common causes of transverse myelitis

Disease	Characteristics
Multiple sclerosis[16]	• Optic neuritis, intranuclear ophthalmoplegia, transverse myelitis, and cerebellar symptoms. • MRI: periventricular, cortical–juxtacortical, spinal, and infratentorial lesions. • Separation of symptoms in time and space. • CSF oligoclonal bands.
Neuromyelitis optica spectrum disorder (NMOSD)[17]	• Optic neuritis and/or longitudinally extensive transverse myelitis. • Recovery may be poor. • Area postrema syndrome can also occur. • Positive anti-NMO (AQP4) antibody (diagnostic).
Acute disseminated encephalomyelitis (ADEM)	• More common in children and young adults. • Typically follows a respiratory or gastrointestinal infection. • MRI: multiple large, confluent, and poorly delineated lesions. • Encephalopathy is required for diagnosis. • Recovery is typically favorable, and recurrence is rare.
Neurosarcoidosis[18]	• Can be bilateral up to 64% of the time. • Other cranial neuropathies, pulmonary involvement, neuroendocrine dysfunction, and transverse myelitis may also occur. • Perivascular granulomatous inflammation. • Angiotensin-converting enzyme (ACE) positive (usually but not required for diagnosis).
Behçet syndrome[24]	• Oral and genital ulcers. • Can cause uveitis and meningitis. • Transverse myelitis. • Common in patients of Mediterranean and Asian descent.
Systemic lupus erythematosus (SLE)[27]	• Rash, transverse myelitis, and neuropsychiatric symptoms. • Anti-double-stranded DNA (anti-dsDNA) and anti-Smith antibodies may be present. • Multi-organ system involvement.
Rheumatoid arthritis[35]	• Arthritis: tender, swollen, warm joints. • Joint stiffness, worse in the morning. • Atlantoaxial subluxation.
Scleroderma[36]	• CREST syndrome (calcinosis, Raynaud's phenomenon, esophageal dysfunction, sclerodactyly, and telangiectasia). • Pulmonary symptoms.

Table 1.3 (*cont.*)

Disease	Characteristics
Nutritional deficiencies	• Deficiency of vitamin B_{12}, vitamin D, vitamin E, or copper.
Lyme disease	• Rash, history of tick exposure. • Multiple cranial neuropathies. • Subacute presentation.

- Partial transverse myelitis causes asymmetric symptoms:
  - Patients commonly present with a hemi-sensory level.
- Table 1.3 summarizes common causes of transverse myelitis.

Intranuclear Ophthalmoplegia and Other Brainstem Syndromes

- Intranuclear ophthalmoplegia (INO) and other ophthalmoplegias are common presentations in MS and NMOSD (Figure 1.2).
  - INO is caused by damage to the medial longitudinal fasciculus (MLF).
  - Patients with INO are unable to fully *adduct the affected eye* when looking to the *opposite* side. The abducting eye usually has nystagmus on end gaze.
  - A common initial complaint is double vision (diplopia).
- In addition to affecting individual nuclei, lesions can involve multiple structures simultaneously.
  - *Bilateral INO*, where neither eye can adduct, can be seen if both MLFs are affected (Figure 1.2).
  - If the sixth cranial nerve and bilateral MLFs are affected, abduction of unaffected eye will be the only movement seen on examination. This is known as the "one-and-a-half syndrome" (Figure 1.2).
- MS can affect any of cranial nerves that control individual eye movements.
  - A Maddox rod can be extremely useful in determining the pattern of ophthalmic weakness.
- Infratentorial lesions can affect the coordination of eye movements, leading to nystagmus, vertigo, and dizziness in about 20% of MS patients.[37]
- Lesions in the vestibular nuclei, cranial nerve 8 at the site of entrance into the brainstem, brachium conjunctiva, and cerebellum can cause a presentation that may mimic vestibular neuritis or benign paroxysmal positional vertigo (BPPV).[37,38]

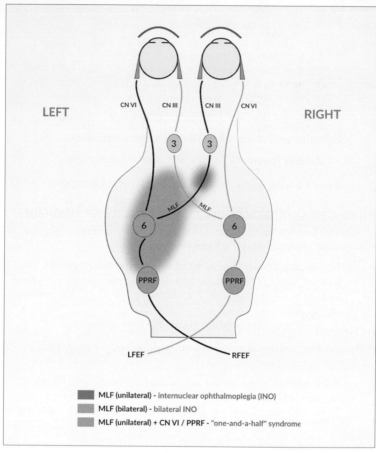

Figure 1.2 Internuclear ophthalmoplegia and other brainstem disorders of gaze. Abbreviations: CN, cranial nerve; LFEF, left frontal eye field; MLF; medial longitudinal fasciculus; PPRF, parapontine reticular formation; RFEF, right frontal eye field. (A black and white version of this figure will appear in some formats. For the colour version, please refer to the plate section.)

- Vertigo in the MS patient can also be related to BPPV rather than to a new lesion,[38] and therefore should always be tested by way of the Dix–Hallpike maneuver.

- *Trigeminal neuralgia* or tic douloureux.

  - Described as a sudden, severe, shooting, electrical pain that radiates down the path of the fifth cranial nerve.

- This pain is typically very brief, on the order of seconds, but can occur multiple times in close succession.
- The pain can be provoked by minimal stimuli such as gentle touch, chewing, or wind blowing over the affected area.[39]
- While the disease commonly results from compression of the fifth cranial nerve by a vascular structure, it can often occur secondary to MS lesions in the pons.
- If trigeminal neuralgia develops in a younger adult or if it presents bilaterally, diagnostic workup for demyelinating disease should be pursued.

Tumefactive Demyelinating Lesions

- The terms "tumefactive demyelination" and "tumefactive MS" are oftentimes used interchangeably. However, they are not synonymous, and not all patients with tumefactive lesions meet the diagnostic criteria for MS (see Chapter 4).
- Tumefactive demyelination is a relatively rare occurrence.

  - The average annual incidence is 3 cases per 1 million people.

- Although tumefactive demyelinating lesions may pose a neurologic emergency, most patients typically do not present emergently to the hospital.
- Potential complications from tumefactive lesions include:

  - Significant edema surrounding the lesion leading to mass effect, which carries the risk for possible herniation.[40]
  - Acute stroke due to vascular occlusion.
  - Seizures due to cortical involvement.[41,42]

- The management of emergent tumefactive demyelinating lesions is similar to emergent management of a CNS tumor with mass effect; it may require neurosurgical intervention and intensive care unit monitoring.
- MRI typically shows (Figure 1.3):

  - Large (greater than 2 cm) lesions with little mass effect and surrounding edema.
  - Open-ring gadolinium enhancement of lesions.
  - The lesions are typically solitary, but multiple tumefactive lesions may occur in some instances.

- Differentiating between a primary CNS tumor and a tumefactive lesion is challenging,[43] especially in the absence of brain lesions typical for MS. In such cases, a diagnostic brain biopsy may be considered.

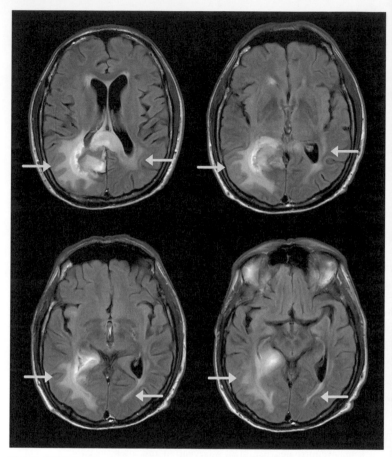

Figure 1.3 T2/FLAIR axial magnetic resonance imaging (MRI) of the brain showing a large tumefactive demyelinating lesion involving the right temporo-occipital lobe with extension into the right hemisphere via the corpus callosum with a little mass effect or edema (arrows).

- Histopathologic specimens of tumefactive demyelinating lesions typically show perivascular infiltrates of mononuclear inflammatory cells with intermingled macrophages.
- The risk of tumefactive MS is increased in patients who are weaning off highly potent disease-modifying therapies, most specifically natalizumab and fingolimod.[44]
  - Close clinical monitoring is warranted when discontinuing these medications.

Indications for Hospitalization

- Most acute demyelinating episodes do not require hospitalization.
- Hospital admission should be considered if:
  - The patient is unable to care for himself/herself at home due to the severity of the neurologic symptoms.
  - The patient requires a medication that can be administered only in a hospital setting (e.g., IV).
  - The patient has a life-threatening infection.
  - The cause of the patient's presentation is unclear and a potentially life-threatening or permanently disabling cause is being considered in the differential diagnosis.
  - IV steroids are being administered for the first time and could cause an anaphylactic reaction.
  - Patient has uncontrolled diabetes mellitus and glucose monitoring/insulin administration may be required.

Conclusion

Most confirmed MS exacerbations can be managed in the outpatient setting. Pseudo-exacerbations should be ruled out by excluding infections. Patients with new-onset demyelinating syndromes require admission unless they can be seen by a neurologist within 1–2 weeks and the symptoms are mild and progressing slowly (i.e., paresthesias).

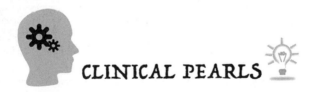

CLINICAL PEARLS

- An MS relapse is defined as a clinical worsening or change in neurologic symptoms that persists for more than 24 hours.
- Pseudo-exacerbations (including Uhthoff's phenomenon) should be considered before diagnosing a true relapse.
- Not every acute demyelinating relapse requires treatment with steroids. These treatments are reserved for patients with symptoms that are severe enough to affect their ability to work or function at home.

- Optic neuritis and transverse myelitis are common ED presentations of demyelinating disease.
- Patients should be hospitalized when unable to care for themselves due to the severity of their symptoms, when they require IV therapy, or when their clinical presentation is unclear and a potentially life-threatening condition may be possible.

References

1. Abboud H, Mente K, Seay M, et al. Triaging patients with multiple sclerosis in the emergency department: room for improvement. *Int J MS Care.* 2017;19(6):290–6.

2. Buckley C, Kennard C, Swash M. Treatment of acute exacerbations of multiple sclerosis with intravenous methyl-prednisolone. *J Neurol Neurosurg Psychiatry.* 1982;45(2):179–80.

3. Dowling PC, Bosch VV, Cook SD. Possible beneficial effect of high-dose intravenous steroid therapy in acute demyelinating disease and transverse myelitis. *Neurology.* 1980;30(7 Pt 2):33–6.

4. Abbruzzese G, Gandolfo C, Loeb C. "Bolus" methylprednisolone versus ACTH in the treatment of multiple sclerosis. *Ital J Neurol Sci.* 1983;4(2):169–72.

5. Barnes MP, Bateman DE, Cleland PG, et al. Intravenous methylprednisolone for multiple sclerosis in relapse. *J Neurol Neurosurg Psychiatry.* 1985;48(2):157–9.

6. Thompson AJ, Kennard C, Swash M, et al. Relative efficacy of intravenous methylprednisolone and ACTH in the treatment of acute relapse in MS. *Neurology.* 1989;39(7):969–71.

7. Miller DM, Weinstock-Guttman B, Bethoux F, et al. A meta-analysis of methylprednisolone in recovery from multiple sclerosis exacerbations. *Mult Scler.* 2000;6(4):267–73.

8. Filippini G, Brusaferri F, Sibley WA, et al. Corticosteroids or ACTH for acute exacerbations in multiple sclerosis. *Cochrane Database Syst Rev.* 2000(4):CD001331.

9. Sellebjerg F, Frederiksen JL, Nielsen PM, Olesen J. Double-blind, randomized, placebo-controlled study of oral, high-dose methylprednisolone in attacks of MS. *Neurology.* 1998;51(2):529–34.

10. La Mantia L, Eoli M, Milanese C, et al. Double-blind trial of dexamethasone versus methylprednisolone in multiple sclerosis acute relapses. *Eur Neurol.* 1994;34 (4):199–203.

11. Beck RW, Cleary PA, Anderson MM Jr, et al. A randomized, controlled trial of corticosteroids in the treatment of acute optic neuritis. The Optic Neuritis Study Group. *N Engl J Med.* 1992;326(9):581–8.

12. Bindoff L, Lyons PR, Newman PK, Saunders M. Methylprednisolone in multiple sclerosis: a comparative dose study. *J Neurol Neurosurg Psychiatry.* 1988;51 (8):1108–9.

13. Alam SM, Kyriakides T, Lawden M, Newman PK. Methylprednisolone in multiple sclerosis: a comparison of oral with intravenous therapy at equivalent high dose. *J Neurol Neurosurg Psychiatry.* 1993;56(11):1219–20.

14. Oliveri RL, Valentino P, Russo C, et al. Randomized trial comparing two different high doses of methylprednisolone in MS: a clinical and MRI study. *Neurology.* 1998;50(6):1833–6.

15. Martinelli V, Rocca MA, Annovazzi P, et al. A short-term randomized MRI study of high-dose oral vs intravenous methylprednisolone in MS. *Neurology.* 2009;73 (22):1842–8.

16. Le Page E, Veillard D, Laplaud DA, et al. Oral versus intravenous high-dose methylprednisolone for treatment of relapses in patients with multiple sclerosis (COPOUSEP): a randomised, controlled, double-blind, non-inferiority trial. *Lancet.* 2015;386(9997):974–81.

17. Weinshenker BG, O'Brien PC, Petterson TM, et al. A randomized trial of plasma exchange in acute central nervous system inflammatory demyelinating disease. *Ann Neurol.* 1999;46(6):878–86.

18. Cortese I, Chaudhry V, So YT, et al. Evidence-based guideline update: plasmapheresis in neurologic disorders: report of the Therapeutics and Technology Assessment Subcommittee of the American Academy of Neurology. *Neurology.* 2011;76(3):294–300.

19. Dudesek A, Zettl UK. Intravenous immunoglobulins as therapeutic option in the treatment of multiple sclerosis. J Neurol. 2006;253(Suppl 5):V50–8.

20. Gettig J, Cummings JP, Matuszewski K. H.p. Acthar gel and cosyntropin review. clinical and financial implications. *P & T.* 2009;34(5):250–7.

21. Balcer LJ. Clinical practice: optic neuritis. N Engl J Med. 2006;354(12):1273–80.

22. Beck RW, Cleary PA. Optic neuritis treatment trial: one-year follow-up results. *Arch Ophthalmol.* 1993;111(6):773–5.

23. Thompson AJ, Banwell BL, Barkhof F, et al. Diagnosis of multiple sclerosis: 2017 revisions of the McDonald criteria. *Lancet Neurol.* 2018;17(2):162–73.

24. Akaishi T, Nakashima I, Sato DK, et al. Neuromyelitis optica spectrum disorders. *Neuroimaging Clin North Am.* 2017;27(2):251–65.

25. Joseph FG, Scolding NJ. Neurosarcoidosis: a study of 30 new cases. *J Neurol Neurosurg Psychiatry.* 2009;80(3):297–304.

26. Gonzalez-Gay MA, Barros S, Lopez-Diaz MJ, et al. Giant cell arteritis: disease patterns of clinical presentation in a series of 240 patients. *Medicine (Baltimore).* 2005;84(5):269–76.

27. Petzold A, Plant GT. Chronic relapsing inflammatory optic neuropathy: a systematic review of 122 cases reported. *J Neurol.* 2014;261(1):17–26.

28. Tang WQ, Wei SH. Primary Sjogren's syndrome related optic neuritis. *Int J Ophthalmol.* 2013;6(6):888–91.

29. Greco A, Marinelli C, Fusconi M, et al. Clinic manifestations in granulomatosis with polyangiitis. *Int J Immunopathol Pharmacol.* 2016;29(2):151–9.

30. Dalvi SR, Yildirim R, Yazici Y. Behcet's syndrome. *Drugs.* 2012;72(17):2223–41.

31. Sedwick LA, Klingele TG, Burde RM, Behrens MM. Optic neuritis in inflammatory bowel disease. *J Clin Neuroophthalmol.* 1984;4(1):3–6.

32. Garcia-Carrasco M, Mendoza-Pinto C, Cervera R. Diagnosis and classification of Susac syndrome. *Autoimmun Rev.* 2014;13(4–5):347–50.

33. McGlasson S, Wiseman S, Wardlaw J, et al. Neurological disease in lupus: toward a personalized medicine approach. Front Immunol. 2018;9:1146.

34. Purvin V, Sundaram S, Kawasaki A. Neuroretinitis: review of the literature and new observations. *J Neuroophthalmol.* 2011;31(1):58–68.

35. Kahloun R, Abroug N, Ksiaa I, et al. Infectious optic neuropathies: a clinical update. *Eye Brain.* 2015;7:59–81.

36. Sharma P, Sharma R. Toxic optic neuropathy. *Indian J Ophthalmol.* 2011;59 (2):137–41.

37. Chavala SH, Kosmorsky GS, Lee MK, Lee MS. Optic neuropathy in vitamin B_{12} deficiency. *Eur J Intern Med.* 2005;16(6):447–8.

38. Sawicka-Pierko A, Obuchowska I, Mariak Z. Nutritional optic neuropathy. *Klin Oczna.* 2014;116(2):104–10.

39. Meyerson C, Van Stavern G, McClelland C. Leber hereditary optic neuropathy: current perspectives. Clin Ophthalmol. 2015;9:1165–76.

40. Klein NP, Ray P, Carpenter D, et al. Rates of autoimmune diseases in Kaiser Permanente for use in vaccine adverse event safety studies. *Vaccine.* 2010;28 (4):1062–8.

41. Sofat N, Malik O, Higgens CS. Neurological involvement in patients with rheumatic disease. *QJM.* 2006;99(2):69–79.

42. Torabi AM, Patel RK, Wolfe GI, et al. Transverse myelitis in systemic sclerosis. *Arch Neurol.* 2004;61(1):126–8.

43. Frohman EM, Kramer PD, Dewey RB, et al. Benign paroxysmal positioning vertigo in multiple sclerosis: diagnosis, pathophysiology and therapeutic techniques. *Mult Scler.* 2003;9(3):250–5.

44. Anagnostou E, Mandellos D, Limbitaki G, et al. Positional nystagmus and vertigo due to a solitary brachium conjunctivum plaque. *J Neurol Neurosurg Psychiatry.* 2006;77(6):790–2.

45. Di Stefano G, Maarbjerg S, Nurmikko T, et al. Triggering trigeminal neuralgia. *Cephalalgia*. 2018;38(6):1049–56.

46. Vakharia K, Kamal H, Atwal GS, Budny JL. Transtentorial herniation from tumefactive multiple sclerosis mimicking primary brain tumor. Surg Neurol Int. 2018;9:208.

47. Yacoub HA, Al-Qudahl ZA, Lee HJ, et al. Tumefactive multiple sclerosis presenting as acute ischemic stroke. *J Vasc Interv Neurol*. 2011;4(2):21–3.

48. Idris AA, Begum T, Verlage KR, Ahmed M. Tumefactive multiple sclerosis presenting with tonic–clonic seizure. *BMJ Case Rep*. 2016;2016.

49. Weinshenker BG. Plasma exchange for severe attacks of inflammatory demyelinating diseases of the central nervous system. *J Clin Apher*. 2001;16 (1):39–42.

50. Algahtani H, Shirah B, Alassiri A. Tumefactive demyelinating lesions: a comprehensive review. *Mult Scler Relat Disord*. 2017;14:72–9.

51. Johnson MD, Lavin P, Whetsell WO Jr. Fulminant monophasic multiple sclerosis, Marburg's type. *J Neurol Neurosurg Psychiatry*. 1990;53(10):918–21.

52. Rahmlow MR, Kantarci O. Fulminant demyelinating diseases. *Neurohospitalist*. 2013;3(2):81–91.

53. Letournel F, Cassereau J, Scherer-Gagou C, et al. An autopsy case of acute multiple sclerosis (Marburg's type) during pregnancy. *Clin Neurol Neurosurg*. 2008;110 (5):514–7.

54. Kuperan S, Ostrow P, Landi MK, Bakshi R. Acute hemorrhagic leukoencephalitis vs ADEM: FLAIR MRI and neuropathology findings. *Neurology*. 2003;60(4):721–2.

55. Hart MN, Earle KM. Haemorrhagic and perivenous encephalitis: a clinical–pathological review of 38 cases. *J Neurol Neurosurg Psychiatry*. 1975;38(6):585–91.

Chapter 2

Clinical Features of Multiple Sclerosis

Carlos A. Pérez, MD

Multiple sclerosis (MS) is a chronic, immune-mediated, inflammatory/ demyelinating disease of the central nervous system (CNS).[1] Although certain clinical features are characteristic of MS, its manifestations can be highly variable among patients.[2] This chapter discusses the diagnostic approach and clinical features of MS, as well as specific features (red flags) that should alert the clinician to the possibility of diseases other than MS ("MS mimics").

What Is MS?

Definition

MS is a dynamic and disabling inflammatory disease of the CNS that is characterized by immune-mediated demyelination within the brain and spinal cord that is disseminated in both time and space.[3] In most cases, it follows a relapsing-remitting course in which the patient suffers from recurring short-term episodes of neurologic deficits.[1,4] Between attacks, the symptoms may disappear either completely or partially.[1] However, permanent neurologic deficits often remain as the disease advances, and a minority of patients experience steadily progressive neurologic decline mostly without relapses.[5]

How Is MS Diagnosed?

A diagnosis of MS is made through a combination of clinical history, neurologic examination, magnetic resonance imaging (MRI), and exclusion of other diagnostic possibilities.[6,7] Other ancillary tests, such as cerebrospinal fluid (CSF) studies, evoked potentials, and ocular coherence tomography (OCT), may be helpful but are often unnecessary.[8]

Etiology

The exact cause of MS is not known, but it likely involves an interplay of genetic and environmental factors.[9,10]

Pathophysiology

Activated mononuclear cells – lymphocytes, microglia, and macrophages – destroy myelin driven by an as-yet-unknown mechanism (Figure 2.1). Antibodies against myelin are also thought to play a role. The pathologic process may be stopped at any time, sometimes after partial remyelination.

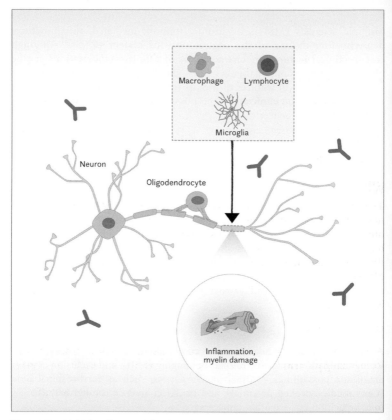

Figure 2.1 Multiple sclerosis pathophysiology. Lymphocytes, microglia, and macrophages destroy myelin by an as-yet-unknown mechanism. Antibodies against myelin also play a role in the pathogenesis of this disease.

Epidemiology

- MS affects more than 2 million people worldwide,[11] including about 1 million individuals in the United States.[2]
- The incidence of MS varies greatly. It is highest among young adults (ages 20–40),[12] but the disease can occur in persons of any age.
- Females are affected more commonly than males, with an approximate female-to-male ratio of 3:1.[13]
- Genetic risk:[11,12]

  . General population: 0.1%
  . People with an affected first-degree relative: 2–4%.
  . Monozygotic twins: 30–50%[11].

    – There is a known association with major histocompatibility complex II (MHC-II) and certain DR2 haplotypes.

- Other possible risk factors:[11,14,15]

  . Geographic latitude (prevalence decreases closer to the equator)[5]
  . Vitamin D deficiency
  . Remote Epstein–Barr virus (EBV) infection[11]
  . Tobacco exposure
  . Obesity

When to Suspect MS?

The *sine qua non* of MS is the presence of recurrent symptomatic episodes of neurologic dysfunction (relapses) that are separated "in time and space."[16] In other words, the diagnosis of MS should be suspected when the clinical history includes at least two episodes of neurologic dysfunction affecting different anatomic locations within the CNS. The evaluation of suspected MS begins with a detailed clinical history and examination. Ideally, MS should be identified based on one relapse in the presence of typical MS lesions on MRI.

History Taking

A complete and thorough medical history is essential when diagnosing MS.[17] Recognizing patterns based on phenomenology and time course is an important first step in making an accurate diagnosis. In addition to the routine standardized questioning, specific information to be obtained includes the following:[5,7,15,18–22]

- Past or present clinically distinct episodes of CNS dysfunction (such as blurred or double vision, weakness, numbness, tingling, gait impairment, imbalance, and bladder dysfunction).
- Detailed chronology of symptom onset during each episode. Typical symptoms tend to occur suddenly or gradually over a few days to weeks, should last for at least 24 hours, and are separated from a previous episode by more than 1 month.
- Spontaneous improvement of neurologic deficits. Symptoms and signs usually disappear within several weeks, but residual symptoms may persist.
- Recurrence or worsening of symptoms as a result of a sudden increase in body temperature (Uhthoff's phenomenon).

Neurologic Examination

A thorough physical examination is critical to localize any neurologic deficits.[17] All systems should be addressed, including cognition, mental state, vision, bulbar function, motor, sensory, musculoskeletal, deep tendon reflexes, coordination, and gait. In addition, a complete physical examination at every visit is necessary to determine any changes in neurologic status and to assess disease progression.[17] Typical signs and symptoms are discussed next.

Characteristic Signs and Symptoms

No single symptom or constellation of symptoms is pathognomonic of MS.[23] However, clinical symptoms stem from neuronal demyelination and loss of saltatory conduction, resulting in slowing of action potential propagation (Figure 2.2). Regular screening for typical signs and symptoms is essential to monitor disease status and progression. Common features are discussed in this section.

Visual Loss

- **Optic neuritis** is due to demyelination of the optic nerve, which typically presents as rapidly progressive visual acuity loss, pain on eye movement, and color (especially red) desaturation. Patients may often complain of a "blind spot" within the visual field corresponding with a scotoma on visual field testing.

  - Acutely, fundoscopic examination can be normal in as many as two-thirds of patients.
  - MRI typically shows T2/FLAIR hyperintense signals within the affected optic nerve. with associated gadolinium enhancement on T1-weighted imaging (Figure 2.3).

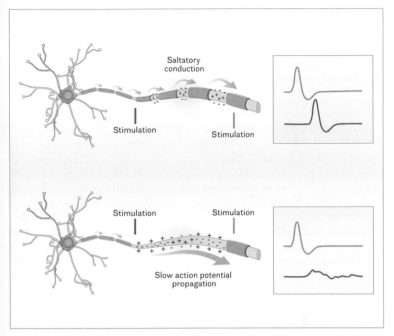

Figure 2.2 Loss of saltatory conduction as a result of demyelination. Linear conduction along demyelinated axons slows because the internodal axon has few ion channels. The loss of myelin insulation of axons allows impulses to spread laterally to adjacent demyelinated axons.

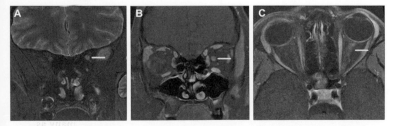

Figure 2.3 Optic neuritis. (A) Coronal T2/FLAIR magnetic resonance imaging (MRI) showing increased signal within the left optic nerve (arrow). (B) Coronal and (C) axial T1 post-contrast MRI showing gadolinium enhancement of the left optic nerve (arrows).

- A relative afferent pupillary defect can often be detected with the swinging flashlight test.[5,24]

- **Afferent pupillary defect** may be due to a current or prior episode of optic neuritis, but may also be present in patients who have not had a clear clinical episode of optic neuritis[5,24,25] (Figure 2.4).

  - When present, an afferent pupillary defect is suggestive of prior optic nerve damage (inflammation) and may be present in patients with prior episodes of asymptomatic optic neuritis.

Eye Movement Abnormalities

In multiple sclerosis, gaze disorders occur when the nerves that control the muscles that allow eye movement are affected. Normally, these muscles work in a coordinated fashion, but when damaged or inflamed, diplopia (or double vision) may occur.

- **Internuclear ophthalmoplegia (INO)**: it is a disorder of conjugate lateral gaze that results from damage to the medial longitudinal fasciculus (MLF) and commonly manifests as diplopia (see Figure 1.2).

  - On examination, **the affected eye** shows **impaired adduction** with inability to cross the midline in association with **nystagmus** in the **contralateral abducting eye**.

Sensory Symptoms

Sensory symptoms are among the most common presenting symptoms of MS and are experienced by almost every patient at some point during the disease. These symptoms are due to involvement of the posterior columns (Figure 2.5), spinothalamic tracts (Figure 2.6), or dorsal root entry zones[3,17,26,27] and may include the following:

- Impaired vibratory sensation
- Loss of proprioception
- Numbness (most commonly of the extremities, but facial numbness can also occur)
- Pain and temperature loss
- Paresthesias
- Trigeminal neuralgia

Motor Symptoms

- **Weakness** affects most patients with MS. Focal weakness is usually due to involvement of the corticospinal tracts (Figure 2.6) and is often accompanied by upper motor neuron symptoms, such as hyperreflexia, spasticity, and an extensor plantar response. Weakness typically worsens

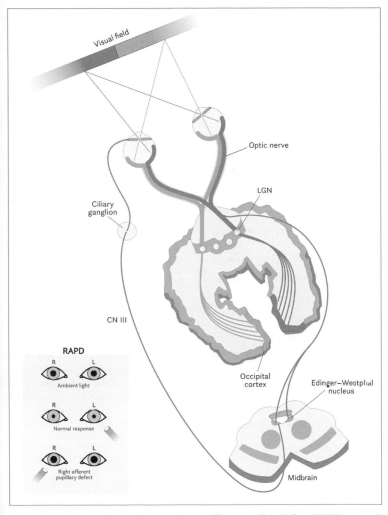

Figure 2.4 Pupillary reflex pathway. A relative afferent pupillary defect (RAPD) can result from inflammatory damage to the optic nerve. A reduced pupillary response to light is seen in which the patient's pupil appears to dilate when a light is shined onto the affected eye. (A black and white version of this figure will appear in some formats. For the colour version, please refer to the plate section.)

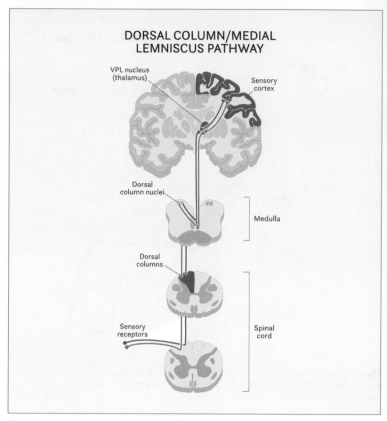

DORSAL COLUMN/MEDIAL LEMNISCUS PATHWAY

Figure 2.5 Dorsal column/medial lemniscus pathway. Inflammatory lesions affecting the integrity of this pathway will result in sensory deficits in fine touch, vibration sense, two-point discrimination, and proprioception. Abbreviations: VPL, ventral posterolateral (thalamic nucleus).

with physical activity.[5,11,28] Bilateral leg weakness with or without a sensory level is often seen in acute, incomplete transverse myelitis – another common presentation of MS.

- **Spasticity** is defined as a velocity-dependent increase in resistance to passive muscle stretch associated with stiffness, pain, spasms, cramping, and gait impairment. Spasticity typically improves with stretching, exercise, or ambulation.[15,29,30]

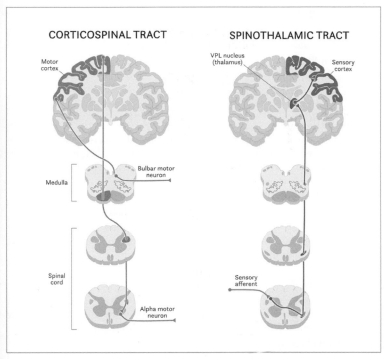

Figure 2.6 Corticospinal (motor) and spinothalamic (sensory) pathways. Inflammatory lesions affecting the integrity of these pathways will result in motor and sensory deficits, respectively. The corticospinal tract controls movements of the limbs and trunk. The spinothalamic tract carries information regarding fine touch, pain, and temperature. Abbreviations: VPL, ventral posterolateral (thalamic nucleus).

- **Incoordination** is most noticeable in the extremities, but slurred speech can also occur as a result of impairment of the cerebellar pathways. Physical examination typically reveals dysmetria, nystagmus, or tremor (most commonly an intention tremor).[5,29,31]

Bowel and Bladder Dysfunction

- Bowel and bladder incontinence may occur.[15,24,32]
- Urinary symptoms include urinary frequency, urgency, urge incontinence, difficulty with bladder emptying, and nocturia.[24,26]
- These symptoms may occur during an acute relapse or may appear over time as a result of disease progression.

Sexual Dysfunction

Sexual dysfunction affects as many as 50% of patients with MS.[1,24,26] Common complaints include the following:

- Reduced libido
- Orgasmic dysfunction
- Erectile dysfunction in men

Gait Abnormalities

Multiple factors can cause gait abnormalities, including cerebellar or vestibular dysfunction, weakness, spasticity, and sensory loss.[24] Typical manifestations include gait ataxia and slowed gait.

Paroxysmal Symptoms

Lhermitte sign is a transient sensory symptom described as an "electric shock" radiating down the spine or into the limbs, most often after flexion of the neck. This symptom can also be seen with other lesions of the cervical cord, such as tumors, disc herniation, and trauma.[17,24]

Heat Sensitivity

Uhthoff's phenomenon is a temporary worsening of current or preexisting signs and symptoms caused by small increases in body temperature (Figure 2.7). This effect can diminish the physical and cognitive function of affected patients with MS.[5,21]

Pain

The different types of pain associated with MS can be neurogenic or non-neurogenic, as well as intermittent or persistent. They include[26]

- Neuropathic pain
- Musculoskeletal and soft-tissue pain (caused by immobility or spasticity)
- Headache

Fatigue

Fatigue is a characteristic finding in patients with MS.[15] It is typically described as physical exhaustion that is out of proportion to the amount of physical activity performed. MS-related fatigue occurs daily and worsens toward the end of the day.[29] On occasion, the onset or worsening of fatigue may precede an acute MS attack and can persist long after the attack has resolved.[15]

A

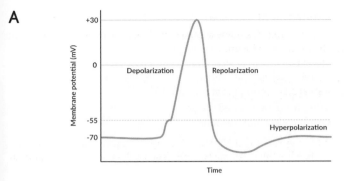

Body temperature increase

B

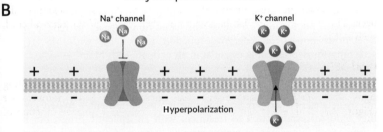

Normal body temperature

C

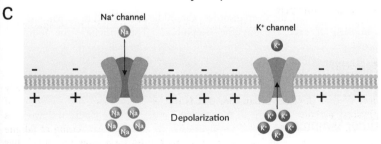

Figure 2.7 Uhthoff's phenomenon. (A) Normal voltage changes in membrane potential during depolarization. (B) Increases in body temperature result in closing of the sodium channel and membrane hyperpolarization. (C) Return of body temperature to the normal range leads to reopening of sodium channels and resumption of normal membrane depolarization.

Cognitive Impairment

Frank dementia is not a common feature of MS.[26] Cognitive deficits are associated with white matter involvement, brain atrophy, and cortical demyelination. This type of impairment usually worsens over time with disease progression and does not commonly occur during an acute relapse. The following domains are most commonly affected:[29,33]

- Information processing speed
- Short-term memory and attention
- Word recall
- Executive dysfunction
- Long-term verbal memory
- Abstract conceptualization

Depression

Patients with MS are more likely to suffer from depression in comparison with the general population.[34] Because this condition appears to have a major deleterious impact on cognitive function in patients with MS, regular screening for depression is essential in all patients with MS.[29]

Seizures

MS-associated seizures are generally benign and transient.[35] When present, they tend to respond well to treatment with antiepileptic drugs, but many patients with this symptom may require no therapy.[5] Generalized seizures are most common, followed by focal-onset seizures with either retained or impaired awareness.[5]

Sleep Problems

In addition to fatigue, sleep disorders should be considered in all patients who complain of excessive daytime sleepiness.[15] These include the following problems:

- Insomnia
- Sleep-related breathing disorders
- Restless leg syndrome

Other Symptoms

Other symptoms can include dysarthria, itching, transient akinesia, and radicular thoracic sensations of pain or tightness in a band-like distribution ("MS hug")[5,24,36].

Table 2.1 Suggestive features versus red flags in the diagnosis of MS

Suggestive Features	Red Flags
Relapsing-remitting disease course	Progressive disease course
Onset between 10–50 years of age	Onset at younger than age 10 or older than age 50
Optic neuritis	Rapid onset of symptoms (minutes to hours)
Internuclear ophthalmoplegia (INO)	Cortical symptoms (aphasia, apraxia, alexia)
Lhermitte sign	Fever at onset of symptoms
Uhthoff's phenomenon	Dementia, seizures
Band-like thoracic pain ("MS hug")	Systemic/multiorgan dysfunction

Suggestive Features versus Red Flags

- A key element in the diagnosis of MS is the exclusion of other possible disease entities that have similar presentations.[3]
- Appropriate history taking is one of the most important methods available for reaching a correct diagnosis (see the History Taking section).
- MS can be diagnosed at the time of the first attack if certain MRI criteria are met (see Chapter 4).
- Certain features (i.e., "red flags") that should alert clinicians to the possibility of diseases other than MS are listed in Table 2.1.
- It is important to keep in mind that none of these features completely excludes the diagnosis of MS, but clinicians should explore the possibility of other etiologies before accepting a diagnosis of MS, especially in patients with atypical presentations or "red flags."
- Atypical cases should be referred to a specialized MS center.

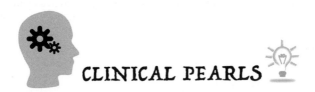

CLINICAL PEARLS

- The evaluation for a diagnosis of MS begins with an assessment to determine whether a patient's presentation is typical for MS-related demyelination.
- A diagnosis of MS is made through a combination of clinical history, neurologic examination, and MRI findings.

- Prior to making a diagnosis of MS, "MS mimics" should always be excluded.
- Atypical features of common MS symptoms – for example, bilateral optic neuritis – may be suggestive of myelin oligodendrocyte glycoprotein (MOG) antibody disease.
- A progressive disease course, rapid symptom onset (within minutes to hours), and signs of systemic involvement (fever, multiorgan involvement) are important "red flags" that suggest a diagnosis other than MS.

References

1. Tillery EE, Clements JN, Howard Z. What's new in multiple sclerosis? *Ment Heal Clin.* 2017;7(5):213–20. doi:10.9740/mhc.2017.09.213

2. Krieger SC, Minneap C, June M, Sclerosis M. New approaches to the diagnosis, clinical course, and goals of therapy in multiple sclerosis and related disorders. *Continuum (Minneap Minn).* 2016;22(3):723–9. doi:10.1212/CON.0000000000000324

3. Geraldes R, Ciccarelli O, Barkhof F, et al. The current role of MRI in differentiating multiple sclerosis from its imaging mimics. *Nat Rev Neurol.* 2018;14(4):199–213. doi:10.1038/nrneurol.2018.14

4. McDonald WI, Compston A, Edan G, et al. Recommended diagnostic criteria for multiple sclerosis: guidelines from the International Panel on the Diagnosis of Multiple Sclerosis. *Ann Neurol.* 2001;50(1):121–7. doi:10.1002/ana.1032

5. Olek MJ. Differential diagnosis, clinical features, and prognosis of multiple sclerosis. In: *Curr Clin Neurol Mult Scler.* 2005:15–53.

6. Filippi M, Preziosa P, Meani A, et al. Prediction of a multiple sclerosis diagnosis in patients with clinically isolated syndrome using the 2016 MAGNIMS and 2010 McDonald criteria: a retrospective study. *Lancet Neurol.* 2018;17(2):133–42. doi:10.1016/S1474-4422(17)30469-6

7. Palace J. Making the diagnosis of multiple sclerosis. *J Neurol Neurosurg Psychiatry.* 2001;71(suppl II):ii3–ii8. www.ncbi.nlm.nih.gov/pubmed/16400830.

8. Carroll WM. 2017 McDonald MS diagnostic criteria: evidence-based revisions. *Mult Scler J.* 2018;24(2):92–5. doi:10.1177/https

9. Mowry EM, Deen S, Malikova I, et al. The onset location of multiple sclerosis predicts the location of subsequent relapses. *J Neurol Neurosurg Psychiatry.* 2009;80 (4):400–3. doi:10.1136/jnnp.2008.157305

10. Brownlee WJ, Hardy TA, Fazekas F, Miller DH. Diagnosis of multiple sclerosis: progress and challenges. *Lancet.* 2017;389:1336–46. doi:10.1016/S0140-6736(16)30959-X

11. Reich DS, Lucchinetti CF, Calabresi PA. Multiple sclerosis. *N Engl J Med*. 2018;378 (2):169–80. doi:10.1056/NEJMra1401483

12. Hollenbach JA, Oksenberg JR. The immunogenetics of multiple sclerosis: a comprehensive review. *J Autoimmun*. 2015;64:13–25. doi:10.1016/j .clinbiochem.2015.06.023.Gut-Liver

13. Hacohen Y, Wong YY, Lechner C, et al. Disease course and treatment responses in children with relapsing myelin oligodendrocyte glycoprotein antibody–associated disease. *JAMA Neurol*. 2018;75(4):478–87. doi:10.1001/jamaneurol.2017.4601

14. Cree BAC, Gourraud PA, Oksenberg JR, et al. Long-term evolution of multiple sclerosis disability in the treatment era. *Ann Neurol*. 2016;80(4):499–510. doi:10.1002/ana.24747

15. Coyle PK. Symptom management and lifestyle modifications in multiple sclerosis. *Continuum (Minneap Minn)*. 2016;22(3):815–36. doi:10.1212/ CON.0000000000000325

16. Marcus JF, Waubant EL. Updates on clinically isolated syndrome and diagnostic criteria for multiple sclerosis. *Neurohospitalist*. 2013;3(2):65–80. doi:10.1177/ 1941874412457183

17. Gafson A, Giovannoni G, Hawkes CH. The diagnostic criteria for multiple sclerosis: from Charcot to McDonald. *Mult Scler Relat Disord*. 2012;1(1):9–14. doi:10.1016/j .msard.2011.08.002

18. Tremlett H, Zhao Y, Rieckmann P, Hutchinson M. New perspectives in the natural history of multiple sclerosis. *Neurology*. 2010;74(24):2004–15. doi:10.1212/ WNL.0b013e3181e3973f

19. Confavreux C, Vukusic S. Natural history of multiple sclerosis. *Brain*. 2006;129 (3):606–16. doi:10.1093/brain/awl007

20. Okuda DT, Mowry EM, Beheshtian A, et al. Incidental MRI anomalies suggestive of multiple sclerosis. *Neurology*. 2009;72(9):800–5. doi:10.1212/01. wnl.0000335764.14513.1a

21. Krieger SC. New approaches to the diagnosis, clinical course, and goals of therapy in multiple sclerosis and related disorders. *Continuum (Minneap Minn)*. 2016;22 (3):723–9. doi:10.1212/CON.0000000000000324

22. Wingerchuk DM. Immune-mediated myelopathies. *Continuum (Minneap Minn)*. 2018;24(2):497–522. doi:10.1212/CON.0000000000000582

23. Thompson AJ, Banwell BL, Barkhof F, et al. Diagnosis of multiple sclerosis: 2017 revisions of the McDonald criteria. *Lancet Neurol*. 2018;17(2):162–73. doi:10.1016/S1474-4422(17)30470-2

24. Gelfand JM. *Multiple Sclerosis: Diagnosis, Differential Diagnosis, and Clinical Presentation*. Vol 122. Goodin DS, ed. Amsterdam: Elsevier; 2014. doi:10.1016/ B978-0-444-52001-2.00011-X

25. Freedman MS, Rush CA. Severe, highly active, or aggressive multiple sclerosis. *Continuum (Minneap Minn).* 2016;22(3):761–84. doi:10.1212/CON.0000000000000331

26. Thompson AJ, Baranzini SE, Geurts J, et al. Multiple sclerosis. *Lancet Neurol.* 2018;391:1622–36. doi:10.1016/B978-0-7234-3748-2.00015-3

27. Miller DH, Chard DT, Ciccarelli O. Clinically isolated syndromes. *Lancet Neurol.* 2012;11:157–69.

28. Polman CH, Reingold SC, Banwell B, et al. Diagnostic criteria for multiple sclerosis: 2010 Revisions to the McDonald criteria. *Ann Neurol.* 2011;69(2):292–302. doi:10.1002/ana.22366

29. Feinstein A, Freeman J, Lo AC. Treatment of progressive multiple sclerosis: what works, what does not, and what is needed. *Lancet Neurol.* 2015;14(2):194–207.

30. Willis MA, Fox RJ. Progressive multiple sclerosis. *Continuum (Minneap Minn).* 2016;22(3):785–98. doi:10.1007/978-1-4471-2395-8

31. Koch M, Kingwell E, Rieckmann P. The natural history of primary progressive multiple sclerosis. *Neurology.* 2009;73(23):1996–2002. doi:10.1212/WNL.0b013e3181c5b47f

32. Sorte DE, Poretti A, Newsome SD, et al. Longitudinally extensive myelopathy in children. *Pediatr Radiol.* 2015;45(2):244–57. doi:10.1007/s00247-014-3225-4

33. Filippi M, Rocca MA, Benedict RHB, et al. The contribution of MRI in assessing cognitive impairment in multiple sclerosis. *Neurology.* 2010;75(23):2121–8. doi:10.1212/WNL.0b013e318200d768

34. Yamout B, Al Khawajah M. Radiologically isolated syndrome and multiple sclerosis. *Mult Scler Relat Disord.* 2017;17:234–7. doi:10.1016/j.msard.2017.08.016

35. van Munster CEP, Jonkman LE, Weinstein HC, et al. Gray matter damage in multiple sclerosis: impact on clinical symptoms. *Neuroscience.* 2015;303:446–61. doi:10.1016/j.neuroscience.2015.07.006

36. Tornes L, Conway B, Sheremata W. Multiple sclerosis and the cerebellum. *Neurol Clin.* 2014;32:957–77.

Multiple Sclerosis Phenotypes

Carlos A. Pérez, MD

The pattern and course of multiple sclerosis (MS) are categorized into several clinical subtypes (Figure 3.1).

Clinically Isolated Syndrome

- Clinically isolated syndrome (CIS) refers to a patient's first demyelinating event typical of MS (e.g., optic neuritis, transverse myelitis, or other common manifestations with suggestive imaging correlate).[1]

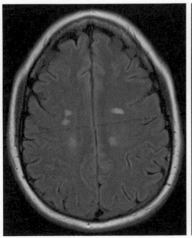
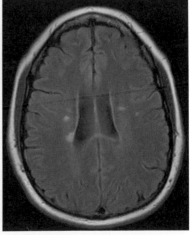

Figure 3.1 Clinically isolated syndrome (CIS). Both axial T2/FLAIR images show periventricular and white matter lesions typical of multiple sclerosis that meet the criteria for dissemination in space (DIS). In a patient presenting with a first clinical event, the absence of enhancing or hypointense lesions on T1-weighted imaging (not shown) does not offer evidence of dissemination in time (DIT). A diagnosis of multiple sclerosis cannot be made on the basis of imaging alone.

- Patients with CIS do not have a history of previous episodes of demyelination.[2]
- Symptoms develop acutely or subacutely with a minimum duration of 24 hours, with or without recovery. Importantly, they occur in the absence of fever or infection.[3]
- Presenting symptoms may be monofocal or multifocal.[1]
- If a patient has normal brain imaging, the risk of future development of MS is about two to three times less compared to a patient with characteristic lesions on magnetic resonance imaging (MRI), but is still in the range of 10–30%.[4]
- If dissemination in time and dissemination in space can be proven by the MRI at the time of the first attack, the diagnosis of MS can be made by the 2017 McDonald MS diagnostic criteria[5] (see Chapter 4). Otherwise, a diagnosis of CIS is given (Figure 3.1).

Relapsing-Remitting MS

- Relapsing-remitting MS (RRMS) is the most common MS phenotype, accounting for approximately 85–90% of cases at onset[6] (Figure 3.2).
- RRMS is characterized by a series of clinical attacks (known as relapses or exacerbations) with full recovery or residual deficits upon recovery.[7]
- Symptoms may last from days to months.[8]
- Minimal disease progression occurs between relapses.[8]
- If untreated, as many as 50% of patients will progress to the secondary progressive phase within 10 years.[6]

  - Recent studies show that this number is reduced when treatment is started early on in the course of the disease.[9]

- At any given time, RRMS can be further characterized into two categories:[5]

  - Active (relapses and/or evidence of new MRI activity) or not active

    - Histologically, acute MS lesions (or plaques) are characterized by the presence of a perivascular lymphocytic infiltrate consisting of T cells and B cells, as well as accumulation of numerous macrophages clustered at the advancing plaque edge containing early and late myelin degradation products.[8]

  - Worsening (confirmed increase in disability over time following a relapse) or not worsening[9]

Secondary Progressive MS

- Secondary progressive MS (SPMS) is characterized by insidious, gradual neurologic worsening with or without occasional relapses, minor remissions, and plateaus[8] (Figure 3.2).

Figure 3.2 Multiple sclerosis types. Relapsing-remitting MS (RRMS) is characterized by relapses or exacerbations that may persist for a short period of time (days to months) with periods of normal neurologic function in-between. RRMS may advance to secondary progressive MS (SPMS), which is characterized by a slow, steady progression of symptoms and neurologic decline. Primary progressive MS (PPMS) is characterized by a slow, steady progression of symptoms and disability accumulation from the onset.

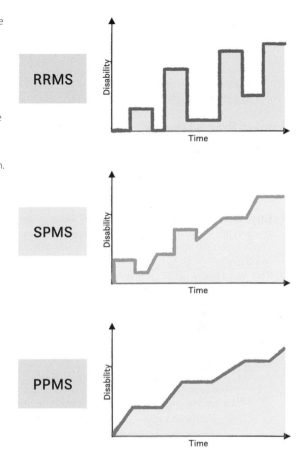

- There are no established criteria for determining when RRMS converts to SPMS, but a diagnosis of SPMS is made retrospectively based on clinical history.[9]
- In most patients, the transition from RRMS to SPMS occurs 10–20 years after the onset of symptoms.[10]
- Since acute inflammatory changes are not as prominent in SPMS, anti-inflammatory drugs are not as effective in relieving patients' symptoms.[11]

- At any given time, SPMS can be further characterized into three categories:[5]

  - Active (relapses and/or evidence of new MRI activity) with or without progression
  - Not active with progression
  - Not active without progression (stable)

Primary Progressive MS

- Primary progressive MS (PPMS) is the least common clinical MS phenotype. It is characterized by progressive neurologic deterioration and disability accumulation from the onset of symptoms without any relapses, plateaus, or temporary improvements[12] (Figure 3.2).
- Clinical findings that distinguish PPMS from other MS phenotypes include gradual spastic paraparesis (asymmetric), predilection for spinal cord involvement (on MRI), and no history of relapses.[13]
- The diagnosis is made exclusively on patient history.[13]
- The median age of patients with PPMS typically ranges between 40 and 60 years, and males and females tend to be affected equally.[12]
- PPMS can be diagnosed in patients with the following findings:

  - One year of disability progression independent of clinical relapses *and* at least two of the following[5]:

    - One or more T2-hyperintense lesions characteristic of MS, located in one or more of the following brain regions:
      - Periventricular
      - Cortical or juxtacortical
      - Infratentorial
    - Two or more T2-hyperintense lesions in the spinal cord
    - Presence of cerebrospinal fluid (CSF)–specific oligoclonal bands

- The most common clinical presentation is a spinal cord syndrome that worsens over months to years, typically in the form of progressive unilateral or bilateral lower-extremity weakness, with or without numbness and tingling.[14]

  - Because of this, patients tend to experience more problems with walking and more difficulty remaining in the workforce.

- At any given time, PPMS can be further characterized into three categories:[5]

    . Active (relapses and/or evidence of new MRI activity) with progression
    . Not active with progression
    . Not active without progression

Radiologically Isolated Syndrome

- Occasionally, an MRI performed for a reason other than for evaluation of suspected MS (e.g., migraines) may demonstrate characteristic MS lesions even though the patient has a normal neurologic exam and no previous history of demyelinating symptoms.[15]

    . As an example, if the lesions shown in Figure 3.1 occurred in a patient who had never experienced any clinical symptoms suggestive of an MS attack, the diagnosis would be radiologically isolated syndrome (RIS).

- Approximately one-third of patients with RIS will be diagnosed with MS. The remaining two-thirds will develop new lesions within five years of presentation.[16]
- In all cases of RIS, it is essential to rule out other causes of white matter lesions[17,18] (see Chapter 5).
- There are no consensus guidelines regarding management of patients with RIS, and current evidence does not support initiation of treatment outside of clinical trials at this time.[14,19]

MS Progression: Summary

- The overall disease course in RRMS is characterized by an asymptomatic preclinical phase (RIS), plus a subclinical, clinical (CIS), relapsing (RRMS), and progressive phase (SPMS or PPMS).[12]
- The different phases are not mutually exclusive and often overlap.[12]
- The relapsing-remitting phase is a more inflammatory phase compared to the progressive phase; the latter is characterized by worsening disability despite a decrease in the number of relapses and overall inflammation.[20]
- PPMS is characterized by a fairly steady deterioration in functional abilities over time.[12]
- The transition from a relapsing-remitting course to a progressive one is a gradual process.[10]
- When a patient's symptoms continue to worsen, an important diagnostic goal is to determine whether the worsening is due to residual deficits from

the most recent relapse or to worsening of the underlying disease despite the lack of inflammatory relapses.[9]

- This can be accomplished by a combination of careful neurologic examination and repeated MRI scans.[10]

- SPMS versus PPMS:[21]

  - SPMS occurs in patients who initially had a relapsing-remitting disease course.
  - PPMS is the first phase of the illness since the initial presentation.

- Low levels of vitamin D and smoking are thought to be associated with a more rapid decline in MS disability and disease progression.[22]
- Progressive MS does not respond to most conventional disease-modifying therapies.[2]
- Ocrelizumab has been shown to slow disability progression in patients with PPMS.[2]
- Siponimod was recently shown to slow disability progression in SPMS with relapses.[23]

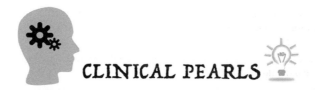

CLINICAL PEARLS

- The different "types" of MS are by no means separate entities in and of themselves. Rather, they occur on a continuum of disease activity – with focal inflammatory lesions at one end, and progressive neurodegeneration at the other.
- Focal inflammatory lesions are the hallmark of RRMS.
- In both SPMS and PPMS, the amount of clinical disability is not well explained by the lesions observed on MRI and occurs independent of relapses.
- Progressive forms of MS are more commonly associated with a motor presentation and carry a worse prognosis with a more rapid accrual of disability.
- Progressive forms of MS are more difficult to treat and currently available disease-modifying therapies are less effective in altering the disease course, although studies of new therapies are under way.

References

1. Miller DH, Chard DT, Ciccarelli O. Clinically isolated syndromes. *Lancet Neurol.* 2012;11:157–69.

2. Thompson AJ, Baranzini SE, Geurts J, et al. Multiple sclerosis. *Lancet Neurol.* 2018;391:1622–36. doi:10.1016/B978-0-7234-3748-2.00015-3

3. Reich DS, Lucchinetti CF, Calabresi PA. Multiple sclerosis. *N Engl J Med.* 2018;378 (2):169–80. doi:10.1056/NEJMra1401483

4. Neema M, Stankiewicz J, Arora A, et al. MRI in multiple sclerosis: what's inside the toolbox? *Neurotherapeutics.* 2007;4:602–17. doi:10.1016/j.nurt.2007.08.001

5. Carroll WM. 2017 McDonald MS diagnostic criteria: evidence-based revisions. *Mult Scler J.* 2018;24(2):92–5. doi:10.1177/https

6. Jones DE. Early relapsing multiple sclerosis. *Continuum (Minneap Minn).* 2016;22 (3):744–60. doi:10.1212/CON.0000000000000329

7. Filippi M, Preziosa P, Meani A, et al. Prediction of a multiple sclerosis diagnosis in patients with clinically isolated syndrome using the 2016 MAGNIMS and 2010 McDonald criteria: a retrospective study. *Lancet Neurol.* 2018;17(2):133–42. doi:10.1016/S1474-4422(17)30469-6

8. Marcus JF, Waubant EL. Updates on clinically isolated syndrome and diagnostic criteria for multiple sclerosis. *Neurohospitalist.* 2013;3(2):65–80. doi:10.1177/1941874412457183

9. Cree BAC, Gourraud PA, Oksenberg JR, et al. Long-term evolution of multiple sclerosis disability in the treatment era. *Ann Neurol.* 2016;80(4):499–510. doi:10.1002/ana.24747

10. Confavreux C, Vukusic S. Natural history of multiple sclerosis. *Brain.* 2006;129 (3):606–16. doi:10.1093/brain/awl007

11. Feinstein A, Freeman J, Lo AC. Treatment of progressive multiple sclerosis: what works, what does not, and what is needed. *Lancet Neurol.* 2015;14(2):194–207.

12. Koch M, Kingwell E, Rieckmann P. The natural history of primary progressive multiple sclerosis. *Neurology.* 2009;73(23):1996–2002. doi:10.1212/WNL.0b013e3181c5b47f

13. Harel A, Ceccarelli A, Farrell C, et al. Phase-sensitive inversion-recovery MRI improves longitudinal cortical lesion detection in progressive MS. *PLoS ONE.* 2016;11(3):1–11. doi:10.1371/journal.pone.0152180

14. Yamout B, Al Khawajah M. Radiologically isolated syndrome and multiple sclerosis. *Mult Scler Relat Disord.* 2017;17:234–7. doi:10.1016/j.msard.2017.08.016

15. Labiano-Fontcuberta A, Mato-Abad V, Álvarez-Linera J, et al. Gray matter involvement in radiologically isolated syndrome. *Medicine (United States).* 2016;95 (13):e3208. doi:10.1097/MD.0000000000003208

16. Alcaide-Leon P, Cybulsky K, Sankar S, et al. Quantitative spinal cord MRI in radiologically isolated syndrome. *Neurol Neuroimmunol Neuroinflammation.* 2018;5(2):1–9. doi:10.1212/NXI.0000000000000436

17. Geraldes R, Ciccarelli O, Barkhof F, et al. The current role of MRI in differentiating multiple sclerosis from its imaging mimics. *Nat Rev Neurol.* 2018;14(4):199–213. doi:10.1038/nrneurol.2018.14

18. Chen JJ, Carletti F, Young V, et al. MRI differential diagnosis of suspected multiple sclerosis. *Clin Radiol.* 2016;71(9):815–27. doi:10.1016/j.crad.2016.05.010

19. Giorgio A, Stromillo ML, Rossi F, et al. Cortical lesions in radiologically isolated syndrome. *Neurology.* 2011;77:1896–99. http://ovidsp.ovid.com/ovidweb.cgi?T=JS& PAGE=reference&D=emed10&NEWS=N&AN=70742614.

20. Lublin FD, Reingold SC, Cohen JA, et al. Defining the clinical course of multiple sclerosis: the 2013 revisions. *Neurology.* 2014;83:278–86. doi:10.1212/ WNL.0000000000000560

21. Ciotti JR, Cross AH. Disease-modifying treatment in progressive multiple sclerosis. *Curr Treat Options Neurol.* 2018;20(5):12. doi:10.1007/s11940-018-0496-3

22. Hempel S, Graham GD, Fu N, et al. A systematic review of modifiable risk factors in the progression of multiple sclerosis. *Mult Scler.* 2017;23(4):525–33. doi:10.1177/ 1352458517690270

23. Dumitrescu L, Constantinescu CS, Tanasescu, R. Siponimod for the treatment of secondary progressive multiple sclerosis. *Expert Opin Pharmacother.* 2019;20 (2):143–50.

Diagnostic Evaluation
Carlos A. Pérez, MD

Although a diagnosis of multiple sclerosis (MS) is mostly made on clinical grounds, laboratory tests and imaging of the central nervous system (CNS) also play important roles in supporting a diagnosis. The value of magnetic resonance imaging (MRI) in the diagnosis of MS is discussed in this chapter.

Diagnostic Criteria

2017 McDonald Diagnostic Criteria

- The 2017 McDonald criteria[1] (Table 4.1) apply primarily to patients with a typical clinically isolated syndrome at presentation and those with insidious neurologic progression suggestive of primary progressive MS.
- The McDonald criteria are useful when the diagnosis of MS is clinically suspected, but they are not intended for distinguishing MS from other neurologic conditions.
- They include specific MRI requirements for the spatial and temporal dissemination of demyelinating plaques in the brain and spinal cord (Table 4.2).
- When used appropriately, the McDonald criteria improve early detection of MS.

Magnetic Resonance Imaging

The diagnosis of MS is based on the principle of dissemination in time (DIT) (Figure 4.1) and dissemination in space (DIS) (Figure 4.2) of CNS demyelinating lesions.[1] Conventional MRI is an essential diagnostic tool in MS, and the main goals of its use in this setting include:[2]

- Identifying typical CNS lesions
- Longitudinal monitoring of disease progression
- Evaluation of response to immunotherapy

Table 4.1 2017 McDonald criteria for diagnosis of multiple sclerosis

Clinical Presentation	Additional Data Needed for a Diagnosis of MS
≥2 attacks and objective clinical evidence of ≥2 lesions ≥2 attacks and objective clinical evidence of 1 lesion with historical evidence of prior attack involving a lesion in a different location	None. Dissemination in space (DIS) and dissemination in time (DIT) criteria have been met.
≥2 attacks and objective clinical evidence of 1 lesion	One of these criteria: • DIS: additional clinical attack implicating a different CNS site. • DIS: ≥1 symptomatic or asymptomatic MS-typical T2 lesions in ≥2 areas of the CNS: periventricular, cortical/juxtacortical, infratentorial, or spinal cord.
1 attack and objective clinical evidence of ≥2 lesions	One of these criteria: • DIT: additional clinical attack. • DIT: simultaneous presence of both enhancing and non-enhancing symptomatic or asymptomatic MR-typical MRI lesions. • DIT: new T2 or enhancing MRI lesion compared to baseline lesion scan (without regard to timing of baseline scan). • Cerebrospinal fluid (CSF)–specific oligoclonal bands (not present in serum).
1 attack and objective clinical evidence of 1 lesion	One of these criteria: • DIS: additional clinical attack implicating a different CNS site. • DIS: ≥1 symptomatic or asymptomatic MS-typical T2 lesions in ≥2 areas of the CNS: periventricular, cortical/juxtacortical, infratentorial, or spinal cord. And one of these criteria: • DIT: additional clinical attack. • DIT: simultaneous presence of both enhancing and non-enhancing symptomatic or asymptomatic MR-typical MRI lesions. • DIT: new T2 or enhancing MRI lesion compared to baseline lesion scan (without regard to timing of baseline scan.

Imaging Techniques

Conventional MRI sequencing techniques used in the evaluation of MS include T1-weighted (T1W), T2-weighted (T2W), fluid-attenuated inversion recovery (FLAIR), and gadolinium-enhanced T1W imaging.[3-5]

Table 4.2 2017 McDonald criteria for demonstration of dissemination in space and time by MRI

Dissemination in space (DIS)

• ≥1 T2 hyperintense lesion(s) in 2 or more areas of the CNS: periventricular, cortical or juxtacortical, infratentorial, and spinal cord.

Dissemination in time (DIT)

• Simultaneous presence of gadolinium-enhancing and non-enhancing lesions at any time or by a new T2 hyperintense or gadolinium-enhancing lesion on follow-up MRI, irrespective of the timing of the baseline MRI.

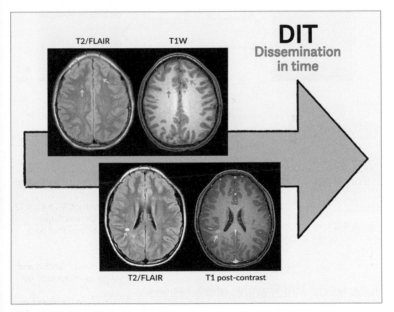

Figure 4.1 Dissemination in time (DIT). The top panel shows both T2/FLAIR hyperintense white matter and periventricular lesions with T1 hypointense correlates consistent with "T1 black holes" (arrows) indicating myelin destruction in the chronic stage of lesion evolution. The bottom panel shows a T2/FLAIR hyperintense lesion that is enhanced with contrast on T1-weighted sequencing (arrows), consistent with a breach in the blood–brain barrier suggestive of active inflammation. Collectively, the presence of chronic and acute lesions meets the criteria for DIT.

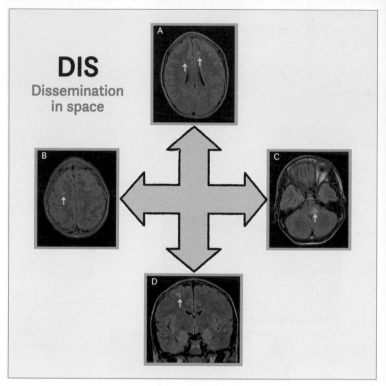

Figure 4.2 Dissemination in space (DIS). The presence of multiple juxtacortical (A, B, D), white matter (A), and infratentorial [brainstem] (C) lesions is consistent with DIS.

Characteristic MRI Features of MS Lesions

MS lesions are focal areas of demyelination associated with pathologic changes due to inflammation, myelin loss, axonal injury, and gliosis.[6]

Lesion Morphology and Distribution

- Classic MS lesions are small, ovoid, well-circumscribed areas that are perpendicularly oriented to the lateral ventricles and the corpus callosum and appear as hyperintense (bright) on T2/FLAIR sequencing.[7–9]

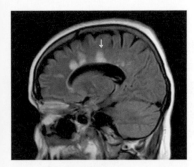

Figure 4.3 Dawson's fingers. Sagittal T2/FLAIR image showing periventricular demyelinating lesions perpendicular to the body of the lateral ventricles.

- When viewed on a sagittal image, these lesions radiate outward perpendicular to the corpus callosum and are referred to as **Dawson's fingers**[10,11] (Figure 4.3).
- Because periventricular lesions appear as bright spots on T2-weighted imaging, they are best seen on FLAIR images, which suppress the bright T2 signal from the CSF.[12,13]
- MS lesions also have a predilection for the juxtacortical regions, cerebellar white matter, and corpus callosum.[14]

Spinal Cord Lesions

- Spinal cord MS lesions are typically small, peripherally located, and are most commonly found in the cervical cord[15,16] (Figure 4.4).
- Longitudinally extensive transverse myelitis (LETM) lesions that extend over three or more vertebrae in length are not typical of MS. Instead, they may raise suspicion for neuromyelitis optica spectrum disorder (NMOSD), sarcoidosis, malignancy, or infection[10,17] (Figure 4.5).

Acute versus Chronic Lesions

- Acute lesions are enhanced with gadolinium on T1-weighted imaging, often appearing in an **open ring** configuration.[18–20]

  - The average duration of MS lesion contrast enhancement is approximately 3 weeks, but about 4% of lesions will remain enhanced for more than 3 months.[21]

- About 10–30% of acute T2 hyperintense lesions can also be seen on T1-weighted imaging as hypointense (dark) areas of demyelination, known as **black holes**.[3,9]
- Nearly half of these lesions will revert to normal in a few months, but as many as 40% of acute black holes develop into **persistent black holes** as a result of severe demyelination and axonal loss.[22–26]

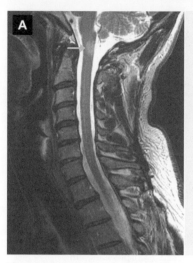 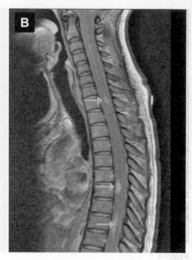

Figure 4.4 Spinal cord MRI images showing a single cervical cord lesion (A) and multiple demyelinating lesions (B) in a patient with MS (arrows).

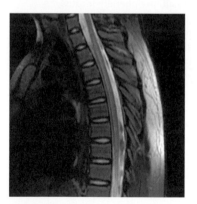

Figure 4.5 Sagittal T2 imaging of the spinal cord showing a longitudinally extensive demyelinating lesion (more than three vertebral segments in length).

Cortical Lesions

- Detection and quantification of cortical involvement in MS using MRI remains a challenge.
- From a histologic point of view, cortical damage in MS has some differences compared to white matter lesions, including a milder glial reaction, a paucity of lymphocytic infiltration, and the integrity of the blood–brain barrier leading to not substantial or quickly resolving enhancement.[27]
- For the purpose of MRI detection, cortical lesions are classified as purely intracortical (accounting for the 85% of all cortical lesions), leukocortical or mixed, and juxtacortical. Nevertheless, standard and advanced MRI techniques such

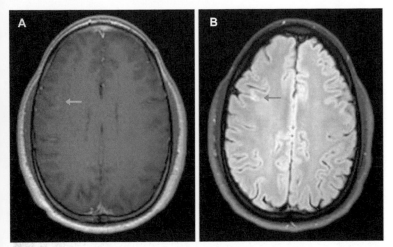

Figure 4.6 (A) Axial T1 post-contrast and (B) T2/FLAIR MRIs showing a cortical lesion (arrows).

as double inversion recovery (DIR) cannot detect the vast majority of them.[28]

- DIR is an MRI pulse sequence that allows visualization of cortical lesions by suppressing white matter and CSF signals[29] (Figure 4.6).

- Information concerning cortical lesion burden is of paramount importance owing to its correlation with cognitive decline and future disability.[12] Although DIR is becoming more widely available, it is not often part of an MS imaging protocol outside academic centers. Nevertheless, detection of cortical lesions is part of the 2017 McDonald criteria, and more centers worldwide are integrating this sequence into their MRI protocols.

Ancillary Tests

Oligoclonal Bands

- The presence of oligoclonal bands (OCBs) in the CSF (by immunofixation and isoelectric focusing) that are not present in the serum is an indication of intrathecal immunoglobulin G (IgG) synthesis[30,31] (Figure 4.7).

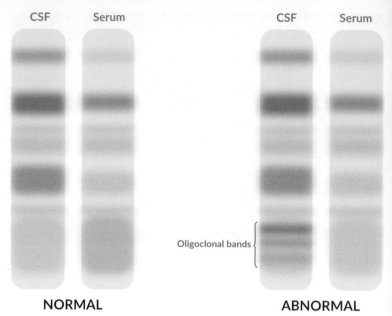

Figure 4.7 Oligoclonal bands (OCBs). Gel electrophoresis showing the presence of additional protein bands in cerebrospinal fluid (CSF) that are not present in the serum.

- Although they are present in the majority of patients with MS, OCBs are a nonspecific finding. They can also be present in other CNS demyelinating disorders and infection.[32]
- When present in patients with CIS, OCBs increase the risk of conversion to clinically definite (CD) MS.[33]
- These markers are especially useful in patients with suspected MS who do not meet clinical and radiological criteria.[32]

Visual Evoked Potentials

- Visual evoked potentials (VEPs) measure electrophysiologic responses to a variety of visual stimuli[31,33] (Figure 4.8).
- They examine a particular waveform (P100) to evaluate conduction along the visual pathway.[8,14]

A

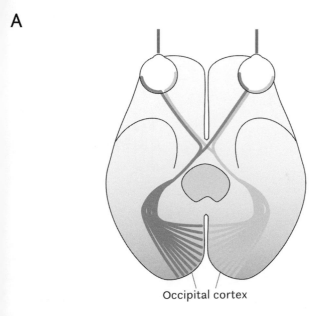

Occipital cortex

B

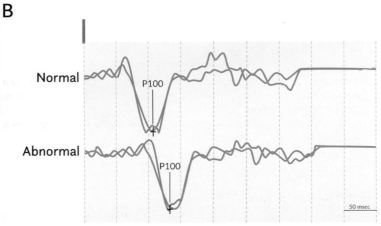

Figure 4.8 Visual evoked potentials (VEPs). (A) A visual stimulus, such as an alternating checkerboard pattern on a computer screen, is given to a patient. The time it takes for the stimulus to reach the occipital cortex (P100) is measured. A delay in electrical signal conduction is suggestive of current (or prior) demyelination of the optic nerve. (A black and white version of this figure will appear in some formats. For the colour version, please refer to the plate section.)

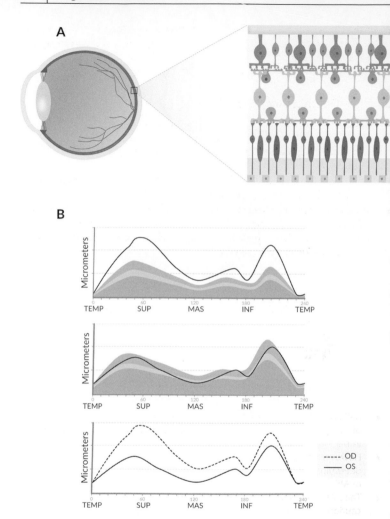

Figure 4.9 Optical coherence tomography (OCT) obtains high-resolution images of the retina (A). Axonal thickness is then measured (B). A decrease in retinal thickness may be suggestive of prior demyelination of the optic nerve. (A black and white version of this figure will appear in some formats. For the colour version, please refer to the plate section.)

- If the latency of P100 between the two eyes is significantly different, this suggests slowed conduction in one optic nerve, which is a sign of optic nerve dysfunction.[32]
- In cases of suspected MS, abnormal VEPs can suggest prior optic neuritis.[31]

Optical Coherence Tomography

- Optical coherence tomography (OCT) uses infrared light waves that reflect off the internal microstructure of biologic tissues, producing images based on the differential optical reflectivity[34,35] (Figure 4.9).
- OCT is used to image the retina at high resolution and to measure the thickness of the retinal nerve fiber layer.[36]
- In patients with optic neuritis, the retinal nerve fiber layer thickness is reduced due to retrograde degeneration of axons secondary to demyelination, which typically becomes evident approximately 3 months after an episode of optic neuritis.[37]

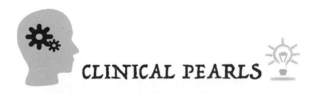

CLINICAL PEARLS

- MRI is a useful tool that may provide objective evidence of dissemination of demyelinating lesions in time and in space that warrants a diagnosis in MS.
- However, as no single biomarker for MS exists, there must always be a determination of "no better explanation" prior to making a diagnosis of MS.
- The 2017 McDonald diagnostic criteria for MS should be implemented with caution in patients younger than 11 years, as they have not been validated in this population.
- The presence of OCBs in the CSF may substitute for the requirement of dissemination in time in the current 2017 McDonald criteria.
- Visual evoked potentials and optical coherence tomography are not required for a diagnosis of MS, but may provide supportive ancillary data for atypical cases in which a diagnosis remains unclear.

References

1. Carroll WM. 2017 McDonald MS diagnostic criteria: evidence-based revisions. *Mult Scler J.* 2018;24(2):92–5. doi:10.1177/https

2. Bermel RA, Naismith RT. Using MRI to make informed clinical decisions in multiple sclerosis care. *Curr Opin Neurol.* 2015;28(3):244–9. doi:10.1097/WCO.0000000000000204

3. Sicotte NL. Magnetic resonance imaging in multiple sclerosis: the role of conventional imaging. *Neurol Clin.* 2011;29(2):343–56. doi:10.1016/j.ncl.2011.01.005

4. Miller TR, Mohan S, Choudhri AF, et al. Advances in multiple sclerosis and its variants: conventional and newer imaging techniques. *Radiol Clin North Am.* 2014;52:321–36.

5. Filippi M, Rocca MA. Conventional MRI in multiple sclerosis. *J Neuroimaging.* 2007;17(suppl 1):3–9. doi:10.1111/j.1552-6569.2007.00129.x

6. Milo R, Miller A. Revised diagnostic criteria of multiple sclerosis. *Autoimmun Rev.* 2014;13(4-5):518–24. doi:10.1016/j.autrev.2014.01.012

7. Granberg T, Martola J, Kristoffersen-Wiberg M, et al. Radiologically isolated syndrome: incidental magnetic resonance imaging findings suggestive of multiple sclerosis: a systematic review. *Mult Scler J.* 2013;19(3):271–80. doi:10.1177/1352458512451943

8. Lebrun C, Kantarci OH, Siva A, et al. Anomalies characteristic of central nervous system demyelination: radiologically isolated syndrome. *Neurol Clin.* 2018;36 (1):59–68. doi:10.1016/j.ncl.2017.08.004

9. Filippi M. Magnetic resonance techniques in multiple sclerosis. *Arch Neurol.* 2011;68(12):1514. doi:10.1001/archneurol.2011.914

10. Geraldes R, Ciccarelli O, Barkhof F, et al. The current role of MRI in differentiating multiple sclerosis from its imaging mimics. *Nat Rev Neurol.* 2018;14(4):199–213. doi:10.1038/nrneurol.2018.14

11. Ge Y. Multiple sclerosis: the role of MR imaging. *Am J Neuroradiol.* 2006;27 (6):1165–76. doi:27/6/1165 [pii]

12. Kolber P, Montag S, Fleischer V, et al. Identification of cortical lesions using DIR and FLAIR in early stages of multiple sclerosis. *J Neurol.* 2015;262(6):1473–82. doi:10.1007/s00415-015-7724-5

13. Zhou J, Tan W, Tan SE, et al An unusual case of anti-MOG CNS demyelination with concomitant mild anti-NMDAR encephalitis. *J Neuroimmunol.* 2018;320:107–10. doi:10.1016/j.jneuroim.2018.03.019

14. Filippi M, Preziosa P, Meani A, et al. Prediction of a multiple sclerosis diagnosis in patients with clinically isolated syndrome using the 2016 MAGNIMS and 2010 McDonald criteria: a retrospective study. *Lancet Neurol.* 2018;17(2):133–42. doi:10.1016/S1474-4422(17)30469-6

15. Kearney H, Miller DH, Ciccarelli O. Spinal cord MRI in multiple sclerosis: diagnostic, prognostic and clinical value. *Nat Rev Neurol.* 2015;11(6):327–38. doi:10.1038/nrneurol.2015.80

16. Alcaide-Leon P, Cybulsky K, Sankar S, et al. Quantitative spinal cord MRI in radiologically isolated syndrome. *Neurol Neuroimmunol Neuroinflammation.* 2018;5(2):1–9. doi:10.1212/NXI.0000000000000436

17. Wingerchuk DM. Immune-mediated myelopathies. *Continuum (Minneap Minn).* 2018;24(2):497–522. doi:10.1212/CON.0000000000000582

18. Chen JJ, Carletti F, Young V, et al. MRI differential diagnosis of suspected multiple sclerosis. *Clin Radiol.* 2016;71(9):815–27. doi:10.1016/j.crad.2016.05.010

19. Klawiter EC. Current and new directions in MRI in multiple sclerosis. *Continuum (Minneap Minn).* 2013:1058–73.

20. Pretorius PM, Quaghebeur G. The role of MRI in the diagnosis of MS. *Clin Radiol.* 2003;58(6):434–48. doi:10.1016/S0009-9260(03)00089-8

21. Khaleeli Z, Ciccarelli O, Mizskiel K, et al. Lesion enhancement diminishes with time in primary progressive multiple sclerosis. *Mult Scler.* 2010;16(3):317–24. doi:10.1177/1352458509358090

22. Filippi M, Rocca MA, Ciccarelli O, et al. MRI criteria for the diagnosis of multiple sclerosis: MAGNIMS consensus guidelines. *Lancet Neurol.* 2016;15(3):292–303. doi:10.1016/S1474-4422(15)00393-2

23. Filippi M, Agosta F. Imaging biomarkers in multiple sclerosis. *J Magn Reson Imaging.* 2010;31(4):770–88. doi:10.1002/jmri.22102

24. Cortese R, Magnollay L, Tur C, et al. Value of the central vein sign at 3T to differentiate MS from seropositive NMOSD. *Neurology.* 2018;90(14):e1183–90. doi:10.1212/WNL.0000000000005256

25. Maggi P, Absinta M, Grammatico M, et al. Central vein sign differentiates multiple sclerosis from central nervous system inflammatory vasculopathies. *Ann Neurol.* 2018;83(2):283–94. doi:10.1002/ana.25146

26. Sati P, Oh J, Todd Constable R, et al. The central vein sign and its clinical evaluation for the diagnosis of multiple sclerosis: a consensus statement from the North American Imaging in Multiple Sclerosis Cooperative. *Nat Rev Neurol.* 2016;12 (12):714–22. doi:10.1038/nrneurol.2016.166

27. Matthews PM, Roncaroli F, Waldman A, et al. A practical review of the neuropathology and neuroimaging of multiple sclerosis. *Pract Neurol.* 2016;16 (4):279–87.

28. Geurts JJG, Pouwels PJW, Uitdehaag BMJ, et al. Intracortical lesions in multiple sclerosis: improved detection with 3D double inversion-recovery MR imaging. *Radiology.* 2005;236(1):254–60.

29. Nelson F, Poonawalla AH, Hou P, et al. Improved identification of intracortical lesions in multiple sclerosis with phase-sensitive inversion recovery in combination with fast double inversion recovery MR imaging. *Am J Neuroradiol.* 2007;28 (9):1645–9.

30. Matute-Blanch C, Villar LM, Álvarez-Cermeño JC, et al. Neurofilament light chain and oligoclonal bands are prognostic biomarkers in radiologically isolated syndrome. *Brain.* 2018;141:1085–93. doi:10.1093/brain/awy021

31. Schäffler N, Köpke S, Winkler L, et al. Accuracy of diagnostic tests in multiple sclerosis: a systematic review. *Acta Neurol Scand.* 2011;124(3):151–64. doi:10.1111/j.1600-0404.2010.01454.x

32. Thompson AJ, Banwell BL, Barkhof F, et al. Diagnosis of multiple sclerosis: 2017 revisions of the McDonald criteria. *Lancet Neurol.* 2018;17(2):162–73. doi:10.1016/S1474-4422(17)30470-2

33. Marcus JF, Waubant EL. Updates on clinically isolated syndrome and diagnostic criteria for multiple sclerosis. *Neurohospitalist.* 2013;3(2):6580. doi:10.1177/1941874412457183

34. Miller DH, Chard DT, Ciccarelli O. Clinically isolated syndromes. *Lancet Neurol.* 2012;11:157–69.

35. Lublin FD, Reingold SC, Cohen JA, et al. Defining the clinical course of multiple sclerosis: the 2013 revisions. *Neurology.* 2014;83:278–86. doi:10.1212/WNL.0000000000000560

36. Zhou L, Huang Y, Li H, et al. MOG-antibody associated demyelinating disease of the CNS: a clinical and pathological study in Chinese Han patients. *J Neuroimmunol.* 2017;305:19–28. doi:10.1016/j.jneuroim.2017.01.007

37. Reich DS, Lucchinetti CF, Calabresi PA. Multiple sclerosis. *N Engl J Med.* 2018;378 (2):169–80. doi:10.1056/NEJMra1401483

Differential Diagnosis

Carlos A. Pérez, MD

Despite recent refinements in the diagnostic criteria, multiple sclerosis (MS) remains a challenging diagnosis. Several acquired and inherited disorders can mimic MS both clinically and radiographically, which may further complicate the diagnostic process. This chapter focuses on the most common diseases that mimic MS ("MS mimics"), the most relevant clinical and diagnostic characteristics suggestive of an alternative diagnosis, and the best diagnostic workup for the exclusion of similar conditions. A discussion of specific magnetic resonance imaging (MRI) features that may help distinguish MS from its mimics is presented in **Chapter 6**.

MS Mimics

Table 5.1 lists common MS mimics. The clinical characteristics of these conditions are discussed in the following sections.

Autoimmune/Inflammatory Diseases

- **Acute disseminated encephalomyelitis (ADEM)**[1–3]

  - **Clinical features:** ADEM typically follows within a few days to weeks of a triggering infection or vaccination. A key diagnostic feature is impaired level of consciousness (encephalopathy). Other typical clinical features include fever, headache, motor deficits, ataxia, sensory abnormalities, seizures, optic neuritis, and transverse myelitis.
  - **Radiographic features:** The pathologic hallmark of ADEM is widespread white and gray matter inflammation with demyelination. ADEM lesions are usually more numerous, larger, and asymmetric, and have poorly defined margins compared to those typically seen in MS.
  - **Management:** Intravenous high-dose glucocorticoids for several days is the standard therapy in the acute setting, followed by an oral taper. Intravenous immune globulin (IVIG) and plasma exchange are also used in patients who do not respond to glucocorticoid treatment.

Table 5.1 Multiple sclerosis mimics

Autoimmune/Inflammatory

- Acute disseminated encephalomyelitis (ADEM), neuromyelitis optica spectrum disorder (NMOSD), anti-myelin oligodendrocyte glycoprotein (MOG) disease, Behçet syndrome, antiphospholipid antibody syndrome, Sjögren syndrome, systemic lupus erythematosus (SLE), sarcoidosis, chronic lymphocytic inflammation with pontine perivascular enhancement responsive to steroids (CLIPPERS)

Hereditary/Genetic

- Leukodystrophies, mitochondrial disease, hereditary myelopathy, hereditary ataxias, spinocerebellar degeneration

Infectious

- Progressive multifocal leukoencephalopathy (PML), Lyme disease, neurosyphilis, HIV, human T-lymphotropic virus type 1 (HTLV-1)

Metabolic

- Vitamin B_{12} deficiency, vitamin E deficiency, zinc toxicity, copper deficiency

Neoplastic

- Central nervous system glioma or lymphoma, primary and metastatic spinal cord tumors, paraneoplastic disorders

Psychiastric

- Conversion disorder

Traumatic

- Myelopathy

Vascular

- Susac syndrome, spinal arteriovenous malformation, cerebral autosomal dominant arteriopathy with subcortical infarcts and leukoencephalopathy (CADASIL)

- **Prognosis:** ADEM is typically monophasic, but as many as 25% of patients may experience recurring attacks. Patients with monophasic disease generally have a good prognosis.

- **Neuromyelitis optica spectrum disorder (NMOSD)**[3,4]

  - **Clinical features:** NMOSD predominantly affects the optic nerves and the spinal cord. Typical symptoms include vision loss, weakness or paralysis of the arms and legs, numbness, and loss of bowel/bladder control.
  - **Pathophysiology:** Autoantibodies against the aquaporin-4 (AQP4) channel are the pathogenic culprits in this disease (Figure 5.1).

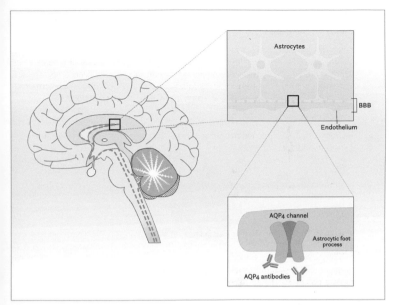

Figure 5.1 Pathophysiology of neuromyelitis optica spectrum disorder (NMOSD). The aquaporin 4 (APQ4) channel is highly expressed along astrocytic foot processes forming the blood–brain barrier within the brain and spinal cord.

- **Radiographic features:** NMOSD lesions are typically large and edematous. Brain MRI may show brainstem lesions. Spinal cord lesions shown on MRI, by definition, are longitudinally extensive, spanning three or more vertebral segments.
- **Ancillary tests:** The detection of AQP4 antibody is highly specific for NMOSD, but antibody-negative NMOSD is not uncommon, especially if the spinal cord lesions are not typical.
- **Management:** Acute attacks/relapses are treated with high-dose glucocorticoids for several days, followed by an oral taper. Plasma exchange is used in patients who do not respond to glucocorticoid treatment. Long-term immunosuppression is typically required.
- **Prognosis:** Recurring attacks tend to be more severe than in MS, with less likelihood of recovery. There is accumulation of disability with each attack, especially if untreated. However, there does not appear to be a progressive phase independent of relapses.

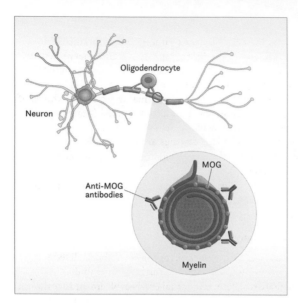

Figure 5.2
Pathophysiology of myelin oligodendrocyte glycoprotein (MOG) antibody-associated disease. Autoantibodies against MOG protein on the outer lamella of myelin are the culprits in this disease.

- **Anti-myelin oligodendrocyte glycoprotein (MOG) disease**[5,6]

  - **Clinical features:** MOG disease commonly presents with bilateral optic neuritis, transverse myelitis, brainstem encephalitis, ADEM, and epileptic seizures. It is more common in children compared to adults.
  - **Pathophysiology:** Autoantibodies against MOG protein on the outer lamella of myelin are the pathogenic culprits in this disease (Figure 5.2).
  - **Radiographic features:** In addition to longitudinally extensive transverse myelitis (LETM), conus medullaris lesions and optic nerve lesions (typically bilateral) are common.
  - **Ancillary tests:** Serum IgG antibodies to MOG protein are diagnostic.
  - **Management:** Acute attacks/relapses are treated with high-dose glucocorticoids for several days, followed by an oral taper. IVIG and plasma exchange can also be used in patients who do not respond to glucocorticoid treatment. In contrast to NMOSD, MOG disease is highly sensitive to oral steroids and requires a low-dose prednisone maintenance regimen with or without immunosuppression.
  - **Prognosis:** Anti-MOG disease is most often monophasic, but a number of patients will experience relapsing disease. A transient seropositivity during or shortly after a clinical attack typically favors a lower risk of relapse.

- **Behçet disease**[3,7,8]

  - **Clinical features:** Behçet disease is characterized by brainstem and cerebellar involvement (dysarthria, dysphagia, cranial nerve deficits, ataxia), hemiparesis, behavioral changes, arthritis, thrombophlebitis, uveitis, and oral and genital ulcerations.
  - **Radiographic features:** MRI can be abnormal in up to two-thirds of patients. Imaging may show focal/multifocal lesions (brainstem lesions are most common), cerebral vein thrombosis, or meningoencephalitis, but these findings are nonspecific.
  - **Management:** High-dose glucocorticoids are used in the acute setting, followed by an oral taper.
  - **Prognosis:** A relapsing-remitting course is not uncommon, and some patients may require long-term treatment with immunomodulatory agents.

- **Antiphospholipid antibody syndrome**[3,7,8]

  - **Clinical features:** Patients have a history of thrombosis, livedo reticularis, thrombocytopenia, and miscarriages in women.
  - **Radiographic features:** Thoracic spinal cord involvement is common. When present, brain MRI findings are typically consistent with ischemic stroke/thrombotic events.
  - **Ancillary tests:** Antiphospholipid antibodies are frequently positive in active disease.
  - **Management:** Acute thrombotic events are typically treated with anticoagulation.
  - **Prognosis:** In recurrent disease, lifelong anticoagulant therapy may be required.

- **Sjögren syndrome**[3,7,8]

  - **Clinical features:** The most common neurologic manifestation is peripheral neuropathy. Though less common, central nervous system (CNS) involvement may manifest as paresis of the limbs, aphasia, ataxia, seizures, vision changes, and internuclear ophthalmoplegia. Other symptoms include keratoconjunctivitis sicca (xerophthalmia), xerostomia, and bilateral parotid enlargement.
  - **Radiographic features:** Optic neuritis may be present in some cases. Spinal cord involvement, if present, is usually longitudinally extensive, spanning more than three vertebral segments. Honeycomb appearance of the parotid gland may be seen.
  - **Management:** Treatment is tailored to the specific organ systems involved. For systemic (including neurologic) disease, long-term immunosuppressant therapy is often used.

- **Ancillary studies:** Tests may be performed for anti-SSA (Ro), anti-SSB (La), as well as Sjögren A and Sjögren B antibodies.
- **Prognosis:** Patients have an increased risk of developing malignant lymphomas.

- **Systemic lupus erythematosus (SLE)** [3,7,9]
  - **Clinical features:** The most common neurologic presentation is neuropsychiatric symptoms. When present, visual loss is typically severe and painless. Other typical features include malar rash, photosensitivity, and arthritis.
  - **Radiographic features:** When abnormalities are present on MRI, they are typically consistent with cerebrovascular disease (ischemic/hemorrhagic stroke, venous sinus thrombosis), optic neuritis, or transverse myelitis.
  - **Radiographic features:** Imaging may show serum ANA and double-stranded DNA antibody. Cerebrospinal fluid (CSF) oligoclonal bands may be present in as many as 50% of patients.
  - **Management:** Treatment is tailored to the specific organ systems involved. For systemic (including neurologic) disease, high-dose intravenous glucocorticoids are used in the acute setting. Strokes are managed in the same way as they are in patients without SLE. Long-term immunosuppression for recurring disease may be considered.
  - **Prognosis:** SLE typically follows a relapsing-remitting course, and the features of the disease vary greatly between individuals.

- **Neurosarcoidosis** [3,7,9]
  - **Clinical features:** Neurosarcoidosis is characterized by cranial neuropathy, headaches, vision loss, ataxia, vomiting, and seizures.
  - **Radiographic features:** Pachymeningeal or leptomeningeal enhancement is most common. Optic nerve involvement can also be seen.
  - **Ancillary studies:** Tests include serum/CSF angiotensin-converting enzyme (ACE) and chest computed tomography (CT) scan, which will be abnormal.
  - **Management:** Treatment is tailored to the specific organ systems involved. For systemic (including neurologic) disease, high-dose intravenous glucocorticoids are used in the acute setting.
  - **Prognosis:** Patients may have a slowly progressive chronic course with intermittent exacerbations. Prognosis with peripheral neuropathy is more favorable compared to CNS involvement. A variety of immunosuppressant agents are used to manage SLE.

- **Chronic lymphocytic inflammation with pontine perivascular enhancement responsive to steroids (CLIPPERS)** [10–13]
  - **Clinical features:** CLIPPERS is characterized by a relapsing-remitting pattern of diplopia, gait ataxia, dysarthria, and facial paresthesias.

- **Radiographic features:** CLIPPERS predominantly involves the pons and typically presents with punctate, curvilinear gadolinium-enhancing pontine lesions on MRI, with variable involvement of the medulla, midbrain, and spinal cord.
- **Management:** High-dose corticosteroids for several days are used in the acute setting to treat acute attacks or exacerbations, followed by an oral taper.
- **Prognosis:** Depending on the severity of the symptoms and response to treatment, neurologic recovery may be incomplete. However, CLIPPERS is generally responsive to long-term glucocorticoid therapy or other glucocorticoid-sparing immunosuppressive agents.

Paraneoplastic and Autoimmune Encephalitidies

- **Anti-N-methyl-D-aspartate receptor (NMDAR) encephalitis**[14–16]

  - NMDAR encephalitis is an immune-mediated disease characterized by the presence of antibodies against the heteromeric NR1–NR2 receptor complex, resulting in internalization and marked reduction of cell-surface N-methyl-D-aspartate (NMDA) receptors in the CNS.
  - **Pathophysiology:** Autoantibodies against the NMDA receptor on the cell surface cause internalization and impaired neuronal transmission (Figure 5.3).
  - **Clinical features:** A viral-like prodrome is typically followed by a multistage progression of symptoms that may include behavioral changes, psychosis, memory deficits, seizures, language disintegration, orofacial dyskinesias, and autonomic instability.
  - **Radiographic features:** Rarely, abnormal hyperintensities on T2/FLAIR may be seen with or without enhancement. Approximately 70% of patients have normal brain MRIs.
  - **Diagnosis:** CSF NMDAR antibody testing is the preferred method of diagnosis. Serum NMDAR antibody testing is less specific, but when possible, both CSF and serum testing may be evaluated.

    - Electroencephalogram (EEG) evaluation may show a "delta brush" pattern, which consists of generalized rhythmic delta slowing with superimposed higher-frequency waves. This finding is not pathognomonic of NMDAR encephalitis but is considered characteristic of this disorder (Figure 5.4).
  - **Management:** High-dose corticosteroids for several days are used in the acute setting to treat acute attacks or exacerbations, followed by an oral taper. Chronically, treatment with immunosuppressive therapy, including rituximab, mycophenolate mofetil, cyclophosphamide, or azathioprine, may be used in recurrent disease.

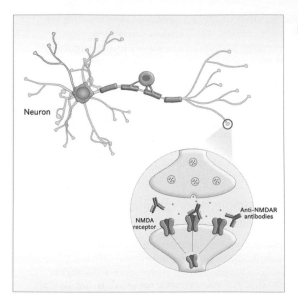

Figure 5.3
Pathophysiology of NMDA receptor encephalitis. Autoantibodies against the NMDA receptor cause internalization of cell-surface receptors, leading to disease.

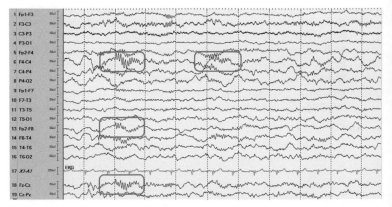

Figure 5.4 Electroencephalogram (EEG) showing a "delta brush" pattern consisting of diffuse delta slowing with superimposed high-frequency activity (red boxes) in a patient with NMDAR encephalitis. (A black and white version of this figure will appear in some formats. For the colour version, please refer to the plate section.)

- **Prognosis:** NMDAR encephalitis is variably associated with ovarian teratomas and other tumors, as well as paraneoplastic syndromes. When untreated, neurologic deficits and cognitive disability may become permanent.
  - Approximately 25% of patients may experience relapses.

- **Anti-LGI1 encephalitis**[17,18]

  - Anti-LGI1 antibodies are directed against the LGI1 protein, which is a secreted neuronal peptide that functions as a ligand for ADAM22 and ADAM23, two epilepsy-related proteins. Binding of anti-LGI1 to these antigens results in neuronal hyperexcitability.
  - **Clinical features:** Common features include memory disturbances, confusion, and faciobrachial dystonic seizures, which may be mistaken for myoclonus or dystonia and are often poorly responsive to antiepileptic therapy.
  - **Other complications:** Patients may also develop hyponatremia and rapid eye movement (REM) sleep behavior disorders.
  - **Radiographic features:** Brain MRI may show medial temporal lobe hyperintensities, as are typical in limbic encephalitis, but is most commonly normal.
  - **Diagnosis:** Diagnosis is made by identification of anti-LGI1 antibodies in the serum or CSF.
  - **Management:** High-dose corticosteroids for several days are used in the acute setting to treat acute attacks or exacerbations, followed by an oral taper. Chronically, treatment with immunosuppressive therapy, including rituximab, mycophenolate mofetil, cyclophosphamide, or azathioprine, may be used in recurrent disease.
  - **Prognosis:** A small number of patients (5–10%) may have an associated underlying malignancy, with the most common being thymoma. Relapses may occur in as many as one-third of patients, and recurrent disease is associated with worse outcomes and an increased risk of long-term epilepsy.

- **Anti-Caspr2 encephalitis**[17,18]

  - Caspr2 (contactin-associated protein-like 2) is an important protein that plays a role in maintaining the normal function of voltage-gated potassium channels (VGKC). Antibodies against this peptide inhibit cell adhesion interactions between Caspr2 and contactin-2, resulting in abnormal neuronal conduction signaling.
  - For the most part, the underlying trigger for this disease remains unknown. However, in some cases, exposure to mercury and other heavy metals has been described as a cause in genetically susceptible individuals.

- **Clinical features:** This disease most commonly affects older men with a median age of 65 years, but rare pediatric cases have also been described. The onset of the disease is insidious, with a median time to nadir of about 4 months. Most patients develop classic symptoms of Morvan syndrome, including encephalopathy, autonomic dysfunction, insomnia, weight loss, seizures, and peripheral nerve excitability.

  - **Note:** Isaacs' syndrome (also called acquired neuromyotonia) is a similar disorder with antibodies against the VGKC complex that is restricted to the peripheral nervous system, and by definition, lacks CNS involvement.

- **Radiographic features:** Brain MRI may show medial temporal lobe hyperintensities, as are typical in limbic encephalitis, but is most commonly normal.
- **Diagnosis:** Diagnosis is made by identification of anti-Caspr2 antibodies in the serum or CSF.
- **Management:** High-dose corticosteroids for several days are used in the acute setting to treat acute attacks or exacerbations, followed by an oral taper. Chronically, treatment with immunosuppressive therapy, including rituximab, mycophenolate mofetil, cyclophosphamide, or azathioprine, may be used in recurrent disease.
- **Prognosis:** Approximately 25% of patients may experience relapses.

- **Anti-AMPA receptor encephalitis**[19]

  - Antibodies against alpha-amino-3-hydroxy-5-methyl-4-isoxazolepropionic acid (AMPA) receptors may cause symptoms of encephalitis in affected individuals.
  - **Clinical features:** This disease most commonly affects females aged 50–60 years. The most common clinical presentation includes limbic dysfunction and neuropsychiatric symptoms.
  - **Radiographic features:** Brain MRI is most commonly normal.
  - **Diagnosis:** Diagnosis is made by identification of anti-AMPA antibodies in the serum or CSF.
  - **Management:** High-dose corticosteroids for several days are used in the acute setting to treat acute attacks or exacerbations, followed by an oral taper. Chronically, treatment with immunosuppressive therapy may be used on a case-by-case basis.
  - **Prognosis:** An underlying neoplasm may be identified in about two-thirds of patients. Lung, thymus, or breast tumors are among the findings most commonly associated with anti-AMPA antibodies. Additional prognostic data regarding relapses are currently lacking.

- **Anti-glycine receptor encephalopathy**[20-22]
  - In this disorder, antibodies are produced against the α-1 subunit of the glycine receptor (GlyR).
  - **Clinical features:** Some patients develop limbic encephalopathy.
  - **Radiographic features:** Brain MRI may be normal.
  - **Diagnosis:** Diagnosis is made by identification of anti-AMPA antibodies in the serum or CSF.
  - **Management:** High-dose corticosteroids for several days are used in the acute setting to treat acute attacks or exacerbations, followed by an oral taper. Chronically, treatment with immunosuppressive therapy may be used on a case-by-case basis.
  - **Prognosis:** Additional prognostic data regarding relapses are currently lacking.

- **Anti-GABA-A receptor encephalitis**[19]
  - **Clinical features:** Patients with this disorder typically develop a rapidly progressive encephalitis with refractory seizures (and potentially status epilepticus). About half of reported cases have occurred in children.
  - **Radiographic features:** Brain MRI often shows multifocal cortical/ subcortical and widespread T2/FLAIR signal abnormalities.
  - **Diagnosis:** Diagnosis is made by identification of anti-GABA-A antibodies in the serum or CSF.
  - **Management:** High-dose corticosteroids for several days are used in the acute setting to treat acute attacks or exacerbations, followed by an oral taper. Chronically, treatment with immunosuppressive therapy may be used on a case-by-case basis.
  - **Prognosis:** An underlying neoplasm may be identified in approximately 40% of patients, with thymoma being the most common. In children, anti-GABA-A receptor encephalitis may develop following a viral disease. Additional prognostic data regarding relapses are currently lacking. Although seizures are typically unresponsive to antiepileptic therapy, patients may respond to immunotherapy and often require pharmacologic-induced coma for prolonged seizures.

- **Anti-GABA-B receptor encephalitis**[19]
  - **Clinical features:** The most common clinical presentation includes limbic dysfunction, encephalitis, seizures, ataxia, or opsoclonus–myoclonus.
  - **Radiographic features:** Brain MRI may be normal.
  - **Diagnosis:** Diagnosis is made by identification of anti-GABA-B antibodies in the serum or CSF.

- **Management:** High-dose corticosteroids for several days are used in the acute setting to treat acute attacks or exacerbations, followed by an oral taper. Chronically, treatment with immunosuppressive therapy may be used on a case-by-case basis.
- **Prognosis:** Most patients improve significantly with immunotherapy. Additional prognostic data regarding relapses are currently lacking.

- **Anti-DPPX encephalitis**[23]

  - Antibodies against dipeptidyl-peptidase-like protein-6 (DPPX) are the culprit in this condition.
  - **Clinical features:** Common symptoms include a prodrome of weight loss and gastrointestinal symptoms including diarrhea and vomiting, followed by the development of encephalitis with central hyperexcitability (including hyperekplexia, agitation, myoclonus, and seizures) a few months later.
  - **Radiographic features:** Brain MRI may be normal.
  - **Diagnosis:** Diagnosis is made by identification of anti-DPPX antibodies in the serum or CSF.
  - **Management:** High-dose corticosteroids for several days are used in the acute setting to treat acute attacks or exacerbations, followed by an oral taper. Chronically, treatment with immunosuppressive therapy may be used on a case-by-case basis.
  - **Prognosis:** Tumors are rare, but B-cell neoplasms have been described in association with this condition.

- **Anti-mGluR1 encephalitis**[24,25]

  - Antibodies against the metabotropic glutamate receptor 5 (mGluR5) are the culprit in this condition.
  - **Clinical features:** Cerebellar ataxia in association with cognitive changes, seizures, or neuropsychiatric symptoms is common.
  - **Radiographic features:** Brain MRI is most commonly normal.
  - **Diagnosis:** Diagnosis is made by identification of anti-mGluR1 antibodies in the serum or CSF.
  - **Management:** High-dose corticosteroids for several days are used in the acute setting to treat acute attacks or exacerbations, followed by an oral taper. Chronically, treatment with immunosuppressive therapy may be used on a case-by-case basis.
  - **Prognosis:** A few patients have developed an associated T-cell thymoma, but most patients have no underlying malignancy. Additional prognostic data regarding relapses are currently lacking.

- **Anti-IgLON5 encephalopathy**[24,25]

  . Antibodies against IgLON family member 5 (IgLON5), a neuronal cell adhesion protein, are the culprit in this condition.

  . **Clinical features:** Patients demonstrate sleep parasomnias (including those in REM and non-REM sleep) as well as obstructive sleep apnea. Other symptoms may include gait abnormalities and autonomic and bulbar dysfunction.

  . **Radiographic features:** Brain MRI is most commonly normal.

  . **Diagnosis:** Diagnosis is made by identification of anti-IgLON5 antibodies in the serum or CSF.

  . **Management:** High-dose corticosteroids for several days are used in the acute setting to treat acute attacks or exacerbations, followed by an oral taper. Chronically, treatment with immunosuppressive therapy may be used on a case-by-case basis.

  . **Prognosis:** This syndrome is most commonly associated with Hodgkin lymphoma, but can also occur in the absence of neoplasia. Additional prognostic data regarding relapses are currently lacking.

Hereditary/Genetic Diseases

- **Leukodystrophies**[3,8,11,26]

  . **Clinical features:** In adults, leukodystrophies can look like progressive myelopathy. Adrenoleukodystrophy (ALD) is characterized by Addison's features, abdominal pain, bronzing of the skin, and family history. Metachromatic leukodystrophy (MLD) resembles progressive myelopathy. In some cases, a family history might be present.

  . **Radiographic features:**

    – ALD: symmetric white matter involvement.
    – MLD: white matter involvement with sparing of "U" fibers.

  . **Ancillary studies:** ALD: serum very long chain fatty acids. MLD: serum arylsulfatase A deficiency.

  . **Management:** Treatment is mostly supportive and tailored to the specific organ systems involved.

  . **Prognosis:** Prognosis varies, ranging from good to fatal depending on the etiology.

- **Mitochondrial disease**[3,8,11,26]

  . **Clinical features:** The clinical features of mitochondrial disease are highly variable. It can present with intermittent, diffuse, patchy muscle weakness, dystonia, seizures, and vision loss, and in some cases the symptoms can be triggered by a febrile illness. When severe, it can lead to multiorgan system failure if untreated. In some cases, a family history may be present.

- **Radiographic features:** Imaging results will vary, but may show white matter involvement.
- **Ancillary studies:** Tests include mitochondrial DNA analysis, targeted gene testing, muscle biopsy, lactate/pyruvate level, plasma amino acids, urine organic acids, and acylcarnitine profile.
- **Management:** Treatment is mostly supportive and tailored to the specific organ systems involved. Pharmacologic drugs with reported mitochondrial toxicity should be avoided.
- **Prognosis:** Prognosis varies, as each inherited disease has its own specific prognosis, which can range from good to fatal.

- **Hereditary myelopathies/degenerative diseases**[1]

  - **Clinical features:** These diseases include a number of inherited disorders, such as hereditary cerebellar degeneration and motor neuron diseases. Typical symptoms include varying degrees of muscle weakness, along with brainstem and cerebellar symptoms. In some cases, they can be progressive.
  - **Radiographic features:** Depending on the underlying etiology, atrophy of the involved areas can be typically seen.
  - **Ancillary studies:** Genetic testing is performed.
  - **Management:** Treatment is mostly supportive and tailored to the specific organ systems involved.
  - **Prognosis:** Prognosis varies, as each inherited disease has its own specific prognosis. In most cases, prognosis is generally poor, progressive, and often fatal.

Infectious Diseases

- **Progressive multifocal leukoencephalopathy (PML)**[12,27,28]

  - **Clinical features:** The symptoms of PML are diverse and depend on the location of brain damage; they may worsen over several weeks to months. The most prominent symptoms include cognitive impairment, progressive weakness, visual, speech and sometimes personality changes.
  - **Radiographic features:** Medium to large hyperintense areas on T2/FLAIR sequences are seen on MRI; they are typically new compared to a previous scan, with or without enhancement. PML is a complication of prolonged use of some disease-modifying therapies for MS, such as natalizumab.

- **Ancillary studies:** Tests seek to detect the JC virus in spinal fluid. Brain biopsy can help confirm a diagnosis, but it is rarely performed.
- **Management:** Plasma exchange is typically used to remove the therapeutic agent involved. No treatment has been shown to be successful, but PML tends to be nonfatal in MS, unlike in other immunosuppressed states such as acquired immunodeficiency syndrome (AIDS).
- **Prognosis:** The progression of deficits can lead to life-threatening disability and death, especially if untreated.

- **Neurosyphilis**[12,27,28]

  - **Clinical features:** These features vary depending on the temporal stage of the disease and the corresponding area of the nervous system affected. Signs or symptoms can include meningismus, vision changes, hearing loss, tinnitus, and tabes dorsalis (sensory ataxia, lancinating neuropathic pain, urinary incontinence).
  - **Radiographic features:** MRI findings may include leptomeningeal enhancement, cerebral atrophy, or T2-weighted hyperintensities in the dorsal columns of the spinal cord.
  - **Ancillary studies:** CSF-VDRL or CSF FTA-ABS tests are performed.
  - **Management:** Treatment consists of intravenous penicillin-based antibiotics.
  - **Prognosis:** Prognosis is generally good unless the disease is associated with nonreversible changes, such as cerebral infarction or atrophy.

- **Human immunodeficiency virus (HIV)**[8,10,28]

  - **Clinical features:** CNS manifestations occur secondary to a direct consequence of the HIV virus itself, opportunistic infections, or neoplasms. Neurocognitive disorders or vacuolar myelopathy presenting with progressive lower-extremity weakness and sensory disturbances, impotence, and urinary frequency/urgency are most commonly reported.
  - **Radiographic features:** Possible findings may include confluent or patchy symmetric periventricular and deep white matter T2 hyperintensities, spinal cord atrophy (most commonly thoracic), and bilateral symmetric dorsal column involvement.
  - **Ancillary studies:** HIV-1/-2 testing is performed.
  - **Management:** Treatment is primarily supportive, with viral control tailored to the individual patient's medical and viral history.
  - **Prognosis:** Prognosis varies depending on the degree of nervous system involvement and viral control.

- **Human T-lymphotropic virus type 1 (HTLV-1) myelopathy (tropical spastic paralysis)**[8,10,28]

  - **Clinical features:** This disease is characterized by slowly progressive chronic spastic paraparesis with bowel and bladder dysfunction and lower limb sensory disturbance.
  - **Radiographic features:** Thoracic spinal cord atrophy and increased signals in the lateral columns, mostly involving the white matter, are common. Cord swelling and peripheral contrast enhancement may also be seen.
  - **Ancillary studies:** HTLV-1 antibodies can be found both in the serum and CSF.
  - **Management:** The mainstay of treatment is immune modulation with glucocorticoids and plasmapheresis.
  - **Prognosis:** The acute subtype typically carries a poor prognosis, with death following within one year of onset, whereas the chronic subtype has a relatively good prognosis.

Metabolic Diseases

- **Vitamin B$_{12}$ deficiency**[1,3,11]

  - **Clinical features:** This deficiency is characterized by upper and lower limb paresthesias, sensory ataxia, gait difficulties, and a swollen tongue. Patients may also have loss of vibration and proprioception in the upper and lower limbs and distal muscle weakness.
  - **Radiographic features:** Imaging shows symmetric bilateral increased T2 signals within the dorsal columns, most commonly involving the upper thoracic region.
  - **Ancillary studies:** Serum vitamin B$_{12}$ level is performed. Some patients with vitamin B$_{12}$ deficiency will have normal serum cobalamin levels. In patients with borderline low cobalamin levels, and particularly in those patients strongly suspected of vitamin B$_{12}$ deficiency, methylmalonic acid and homocysteine levels should be checked. Methylmalonic acid and homocysteine levels are increased in as many as one-third of patients with low–normal serum cobalamin levels
  - **Management:** Treatment consists of vitamin B$_{12}$ replacement.
  - **Prognosis:** Approximately half of all affected patients will completely recover.

- **Vitamin E deficiency**[1,3,11]

  - **Clinical and radiographic features:** These features may be indistinguishable from those associated with vitamin B$_{12}$ deficiency.
  - **Ancillary studies:** Serum vitamin E level is performed.
  - **Management:** Treatment consists of vitamin E replacement.
  - **Prognosis:** Prognosis is typically excellent with appropriate treatment.

- **Zinc toxicity**[1,3,11]
    - **Clinical features:** Patients experience acute nausea and vomiting. This condition can also present subacutely with loss of vibration and proprioception in the upper and lower limb, sensory gait ataxia, and distal muscle weakness.
    - **Radiographic features:** Imaging shows symmetric bilateral increased T2 signals within the dorsal columns of the spinal cord.
    - **Ancillary studies:** Serum zinc level is performed.
    - **Management:** Treatment is supportive; copper supplementation may be considered.
    - **Prognosis:** Most patients recover with adequate treatment.

- **Copper deficiency**[1,3,11]
    - **Clinical features:** Patients experience loss of vibration and proprioception in the upper and lower limb, sensory gait ataxia, and distal muscle weakness.
    - **Radiographic features:** Imaging shows symmetric bilateral increased T2 signals within the dorsal columns of the spinal cord.
    - **Ancillary studies:** Serum copper level is performed.
    - **Management:** Treatment consists of copper supplementation.
    - **Prognosis:** A majority of patients recover with appropriate treatment.

Neoplastic Disease
- **Primary CNS tumors (lymphoma)**[3,7]
    - **Clinical features:** Symptoms include increased intracranial pressure, focal muscle weakness, sensory disturbances, and seizures.
    - **Radiographic features:** Typical high-grade tumors may show homogeneous enhancement, whereas peripheral ring lesion enhancement may be seen in immunocompromised patients.
    - **Management:** Treatment typically consists of a combination of chemotherapy, radiation therapy, and, when clinically indicated, high-dose corticosteroids.
    - **Prognosis:** Prognosis is highly variable; recurrent cases are associated with a poor prognosis.

- **Paraneoplastic disorders**[3,7]
    - **Clinical features:** These disorders are characterized by gait unsteadiness, dysarthria, diplopia, dysphagia, weight loss, and fever.

- **Radiographic features:** In some cases, cerebellar atrophy may be seen.
- **Ancillary studies:** Positive anti-Yo, anti-Hu, and anti-Tr tests are most frequently associated with paraneoplastic disorders. CSF protein is typically elevated.
- **Management:** Treatment depends on the specific cause.
- **Prognosis:** Prognosis is highly variable and depends on the specific cause.

Psychiatric Conditions

- **Conversion disorder**[29]

  - **Clinical features:** Symptoms can include blindness, paralysis, decreased sensation, fatigue, dizziness, vertigo, and pain.
  - **Radiographic features:** MRI evaluation is normal.
  - **Management:** Treatment consists of psychotherapy and cognitive-behavioral therapy.
  - **Prognosis:** Most individuals improve over time.

Trauma

- **Myelopathy**[9]

  - **Clinical features:** Patients may experience weakness, spasticity, hyperreflexia, sensory deficits, bowel/bladder symptoms, and sexual dysfunction.
  - **Radiographic features:** These features depend on the location, cause, and extent of injury or trauma.
  - **Management:** Treatment is based on the inciting event.
  - **Prognosis:** Prognosis varies, depending on the extent of injury.

Vascular Disease

- **Susac syndrome**[30]

  - **Clinical features:** This syndrome is characterized by behavioral disturbances, cognitive impairment, ataxia, dysarthria, headache, hearing loss, vision changes, and focal neurologic deficits.
  - **Radiographic features:** Imaging shows rounded T2 hyperintense "snowball" lesions with involvement of the corpus callosum. Leptomeningeal and gray matter enhancement may be present.
  - **Ancillary studies:** Tests may include an audiogram and fundoscopic exam.
  - **Management:** Glucocorticoids can be used in the acute setting.
  - **Prognosis:** Susac syndrome most commonly presents as a monophasic and self-limiting condition, but some patients may

have residual neurological sequelae, especially related to retinal infarction.

- **Spinal arteriovenous malformation (AVM)**[11]

  - **Clinical features:** These features vary, but may include weakness, spasticity, hyperreflexia, sensory deficits, bowel/bladder symptoms, and sexual dysfunction. The acuity of symptoms can range from progressive myelopathy to acute spinal hemorrhage.
  - **Radiographic features:** Imaging shows signal voids from high-velocity flow, with increased T2 signals from cytotoxic edema or myelomalacia.
  - **Management:** Surgery and angioembolization have a role in treatment of AVM.
  - **Prognosis:** Prognosis depends on the location and extent of injury (including nonreversible injury).

- **Cerebral autosomal dominant arteriopathy with subcortical infarcts and leukoencephalopathy (CADASIL)**[10]

  - **Clinical features:** Patients have headache and stroke-like episodes. Family history of stroke is common.
  - **Radiographic features:** Imaging shows diffuse white matter changes, with anterior temporal and external capsule involvement.
  - **Ancillary studies:** NOTCH3 gene testing is appropriate.
  - **Management:** Treatment is mostly supportive, with an emphasis on secondary stroke prevention.
  - **Prognosis:** CADASIL typically follows a variable but progressive course, leading to death between 50 and 70 years of age.

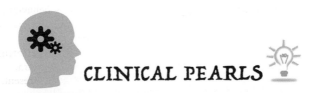

CLINICAL PEARLS

- MS mimics, which include a number of inflammatory, infectious, metabolic, genetic, and neoplastic entities, must be ruled out prior to making a diagnosis of MS.

- Having MS by no means excludes the possibility of having another illness, which further emphasizes the importance of considering alternative diagnoses.
- Migraine and chronic cerebrovascular disease are some of the most commonly encountered MS mimics. However, a thorough review of MRI results can help achieve a correct diagnosis.
- When conversion or somatization disorder is suspected in a patient, clinical depression should be ruled out.
- One of the most common reasons for misdiagnosis in MS and its mimics is MRI misinterpretation. Therefore, a thorough medical history and, when necessary, ancillary testing – including visual evoked responses and optical coherence tomography – can facilitate the diagnostic process.

References

1. Tornes L, Conway B, Sheremata W. Multiple sclerosis and the cerebellum. *Neurol Clin*. 2014;32:957–77.

2. Baumann M, Grams A, Djurdjevic T, et al. MRI of the first event in pediatric acquired demyelinating syndromes with antibodies to myelin oligodendrocyte glycoprotein. *J Neurol*. 2018;265(4):845–55. doi:10.1007/s00415-018-8781-3

3. Renowden S. Imaging in multiple sclerosis and related disorders. *Pract Neurol*. 2014;14(5):1–20. doi:10.1136/practneurol-2014-000856

4. Takewaki D, Lin Y, Sato W, et al. Normal brain imaging accompanies neuroimmunologically justified, autoimmune encephalomyelitis. *Neurol Neuroimmunol Neuroinflammation*. 2018;5:e456. doi:10.1212/ NXI.0000000000000456

5. Adoni T. Anti-MOG syndrome: a road to be paved. *Arq Neuropsiquiatr*. 2017;75(10):685–6. doi:10.1212/NXI.0000000000000081

6. Nakamura Y, Nakajima H, Tani H, et al. Anti-MOG antibody-positive ADEM following infectious mononucleosis due to a primary EBV infection: a case report. *BMC Neurol*. 2017;17(1):76. doi:10.1186/s12883-017-0858-6

7. Wingerchuk DM. Immune-mediated myelopathies. *Continuum (Minneap Minn)*. 2018;24(2):497–22. doi:10.1212/CON.0000000000000582

8. Gelfand JM.*Multiple Sclerosis: Diagnosis, Differential Diagnosis, and Clinical Presentation*. Vol 122. Goodin DS, ed. Amsterdam: Elsevier; 2014. doi:10.1016/ B978-0-444-52001-2.00011-X.

9. Bou-Haidar P, Peduto A, Karunaratne N. Differential diagnosis of T2 hyperintense spinal cord lesions: Part B. *J Med Imaging Radiat Oncol.* 2009;53(2):152–9. doi:10.1111/j.1754-9485.2009.02067.x

10. Brownlee WJ, Hardy TA, Fazekas F, Miller DH. Diagnosis of multiple sclerosis: progress and challenges. *Lancet.* 2017;389:1336–46. doi:10.1016/S0140-6736(16) 30959-X

11. Rostasy K, Bajer-Kornek B, Venkateswaran S, et al. Differential diagnosis and evaluation in pediatric inflammatory demyelinating disorders. *Neurology.* 2016;87(9 suppl 2):S28–37.

12. Balashov K. Imaging of central nervous system demyelinating disorders. *Continuum (Minneap Minn).* 2016;22(5):1613–35. doi:10.1212/ CON.0000000000000373

13. Thompson AJ, Baranzini SE, Geurts J, et al. Multiple sclerosis. *Lancet Neurol.* 2018;391:1622–36. doi:10.1016/B978-0-7234-3748-2.00015-3

14. Yu S, Ran Y, Dong Z, et al. Anti-NMDAR encephalitis followed by seropositive neuromyelitis optica spectrum disorder: a case report and literature review. *Clin Neurol Neurosurg.* 2017;155:75–82. doi:10.1016/j.clineuro.2017.02.016

15. Pérez CA, Agyei P, Gogia B, et al. Overlapping autoimmune syndrome: a case of concomitant anti-NMDAR encephalitis and myelin oligodendrocyte glycoprotein (MOG) antibody disease. *J Neuroimmunol.* 2020;339. doi:10.1016/j. jneuroim.2019.577124

16. Baheerathan A, Brownlee WJ, Chard DT, et al. Antecedent anti-NMDA receptor encephalitis in two patients with multiple sclerosis. *Mult Scler Relat Disord.* 2017;12:20–2. doi:10.1016/j.msard.2016.12.009

17. Sharma A, Kaur M, Paul M. Morvan's syndrome with anti contactin associated protein like 2-voltage gated potassium channel antibody presenting with syndrome of inappropriate antidiuretic hormone secretion. *J Neurosci Rural Pract.* 2016;7(4):577–9. doi:10.4103/0976-3147.188638

18. Nosadini M, Toldo I, Tascini B, et al. LGI1 and CASPR2 autoimmunity in children: systematic literature review and report of a young girl with Morvan syndrome. *J Neuroimmunol.* 2019;335:577008. doi:10.1016/j.jneuroim.2019.577008

19. Kleopa KA. Autoimmune channelopathies of the nervous system. *Curr Neuropharmacol.* 2011;9(3):458–67. doi:10.2174/157015911796557966

20. Huang K, Luo YB, Yang H. Autoimmune channelopathies at neuromuscular junction. *Front Neurol.* 2019;10:1–16. doi:10.3389/fneur.2019.00516

21. Bien CI, Nehls F, Kollmar R, et al. Identification of adenylate kinase 5 antibodies during routine diagnostics in a tissue-based assay: three new cases and a review of the literature. *J Neuroimmunol.* 2019;334. doi:10.1016/j.jneuroim.2019.576975

22. Lancaster E, Dalmau J. Neuronal autoantigens: pathogenesis, associated disorders and antibody testing. *Nat Rev Neurol.* 2012;8(7):380–90. doi:10.1038/nrneurol.2012.99

23. Hara M, Ariño H, Petit-Pedrol M, et al. DPPX antibody-associated encephalitis: main syndrome and antibody effects. *Neurology.* 2017;88(14):1340.

24. Abrantes F, Toso FF, Povoas OG, Hoftberger R. Autoimmune encephalitis: a review of diagnosis and treatment. *Arq Neuropsiquiatr.* 2017:41–9.

25. Dale RC. Autoimmune encephalitis: overview of clinical recognition, autoantibody diagnostic markers, and treatment of autoimmune encephalitis. In: Yamanouchi H, Moshé SL, Okumura A, eds. *Acute Encephalopathy and Encephalitis in Infancy and Its Related Disorders.* Nagakute, Japan: Elsevier; 2017:123–32.

26. Olek MJ. Differential diagnosis, clinical features, and prognosis of multiple sclerosis. *Curr Clin Neurol Mult Scler.* 2005:15–53.

27. Marcus JF, Waubant EL. Updates on clinically isolated syndrome and diagnostic criteria for multiple sclerosis. *Neurohospitalist.* 2013;3(2):65–80. doi:10.1177/1941874412457183

28. Palace J. Making the diagnosis of multiple sclerosis. *J Neurol Neurosurg Psychiatry.* 2001;71(suppl II):ii3–8. www.ncbi.nlm.nih.gov/pubmed/16400830.

29. Stone J, Smyth R, Carson A, et al. Systematic review of misdiagnosis of conversion symptoms and "hysteria." *Br Med J.* 2005;331(7523):989–91. doi:10.1136/bmj.38628.466898.55

30. Chen JJ, Carletti F, Young V, Mckean D, Quaghebeur G. MRI differential diagnosis of suspected multiple sclerosis. *Clin Radiol.* 2016;71(9):815–27. doi:10.1016/j.crad.2016.05.010

Chapter 6

Neuroimaging in Multiple Sclerosis and Its Mimics

Carlos A. Pérez, MD

Since its introduction in the 1980s, magnetic resonance imaging (MRI) has become an essential tool in supporting the diagnosis, monitoring, and evaluation of therapeutic response in multiple sclerosis (MS). Although MS is mostly a clinical diagnosis, MRI has the ability to sensitively and noninvasively demonstrate the spatial and temporal dissemination of demyelinating plaques in the brain and spinal cord in the axial, sagittal, and coronal planes that are characteristic of MS (Figure 6.1). In this chapter, we discuss basic MRI sequencing techniques and provide examples of common radiographic findings in MS and MS mimics. Note that the list of alternative diagnoses presented in this chapter is not all-inclusive.

MRI Signal Creation

- MRI uses a magnetic field that aligns randomly oriented hydrogen atoms (protons) within water molecules in the same or opposite direction as the external field.[1]
- The alignment is briefly disrupted by the introduction of an external radio frequency (RF) pulse. The excited hydrogen atoms emit resonance signals as they return to their previously aligned state, which are then measured by a receiving coil.[2]
- The frequency information contained in the signal from each location in the imaged plane is then converted to corresponding intensity levels that are displayed as shades of gray in a matrix arrangement of pixels.[3]
- By varying the sequence of RF pulses applied and collected, different types of images are created (Figure 6.2).[4]

T1-Weighted Sequencing

The longitudinal relaxation time, or T1, is the time constant that determines the rate at which the excited protons realign with the external magnetic field.[2]

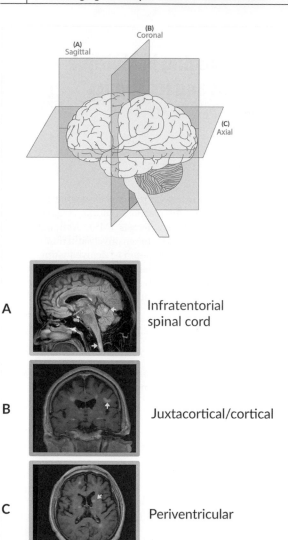

Figure 6.1 Typical locations of multiple sclerosis lesions in the sagittal (A),coronal (B), and axial (C) planes. (A black and white version of this figure will appear in some formats. For the colour version, please refer to the plate section.)

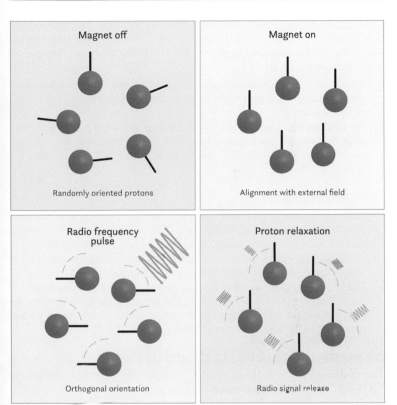

Figure 6.2 Magnetic resonance imaging (MRI) signal creation.

The more quickly the protons become realigned, the greater (and brighter) the signal.

- Tissues with high fat content (such as white matter) will be bright, and compartments filled with water (such as cerebrospinal fluid [CSF]) will be dark on T1-weighted scans.
- T1-weighted images are best for demonstrating anatomy.

T2-Weighted Sequencing

The transverse relaxation time, or T2, is the time constant that determines the rate at which the excited protons lose resonance perpendicular to the main field and become out of phase with each other after being excited by an RF pulse (i.e., dephasing).[1] Dephasing occurs due to random and time-dependent field variations induced by spins of neighboring atoms, since not all spins have exactly the same precession frequency.[1] The slower the dephasing, the greater (and brighter) the T2 signal.[2]

- Tissues with high fat content (such as white matter) will be dark, and compartments filled with water (such as CSF) will be bright on T2-weighted scans.

- T2-weighted scans are a good choice for demonstrating pathology since most (but not all) brain lesions tend to develop edema and/or are associated with an increase in water content, which will make them appear bright.

FLAIR Sequencing

- FLAIR is similar to a T2-weighted image, but the high signal of normal CSF fluid is attenuated and made dark.[5]

- As with the T2-weighted image, this sequence is very sensitive to pathology and makes the differentiation between CSF and brain parenchymal abnormalities much easier to distinguish.[6]

- FLAIR is particularly useful in detecting subtle changes at the periphery of the hemispheres and in the periventricular regions close to CSF, where the high intensity of the CSF signal itself may attenuate visible contrast when compared to the high intensity of nearby lesions.[5,7]

Diagnostic Utility of MRI in MS and Its Mimics

The diagnosis of MS is based on the principles of dissemination in time (DIT) and dissemination in space (DIS) of central nervous system (CNS) demyelination (Figure 6.3; also see **Chapter 4**).

- The activity and formation of MS lesions can be divided into an acute phase characterized by lesional contrast enhancement, and a subacute phase characterized by changes in lesion signal intensity and size on unenhanced T1- and T2-weighted images.

- Gadolinium enhancement may last up to two months in acute lesions, but the average duration is three weeks.[8]

- The subacute phase of MS lesion morphology and activity can be subdivided into early and late periods:[2]

  . In the early subacute period (within the initial ten weeks), the T2-hyperintense lesion is a combination of an influx of inflammatory cells resulting in demyelination, axonal transection, and edema.

  . In the late subacute period (three to five months later), the T2-hyperintense lesion often decreases in size, not only because

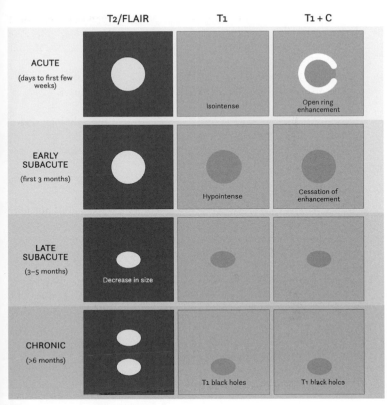

Figure 6.3 Evolution of multiple sclerosis lesions over time. Chronic lesions may disappear on T1 sequencing; those that persist become known as "T1 black holes." Abbreviations: T1+C, T1 with contrast.

of decreased vasogenic edema but also through a combination of degenerative and regenerative processes such as gliosis and remyelination.

. Over the initial six-month period, fewer than 40% of lesions become persistently hypointense on T1-weighted imaging, presumably secondary to permanent demyelination and severe axonal loss. These lesions are referred to as "T1 black holes."[3]

– The accumulation of T1 black holes has been shown to correlate with disease progression and disability.

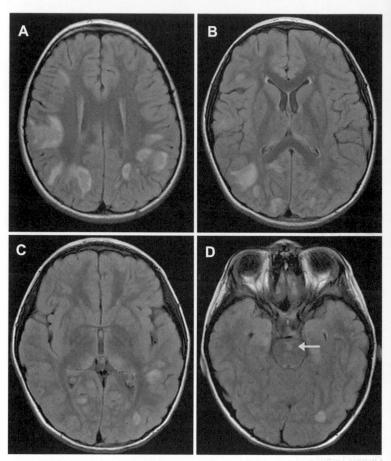

Figure 6.4 Acute disseminated encephalomyelitis (ADEM). Axial T2/FLAIR images show bilateral, diffuse hyperintense lesions involving the cerebral white matter and the pons (arrow).

Autoimmune/Inflammatory Diseases
Acute Disseminated Encephalomyelitis (ADEM)

- ADEM typically presents with diffuse white and gray matter inflammation lesions that are usually more numerous, larger, and asymmetric, and have poorly defined margins compared to the lesions typically seen in MS (Figure 6.4).

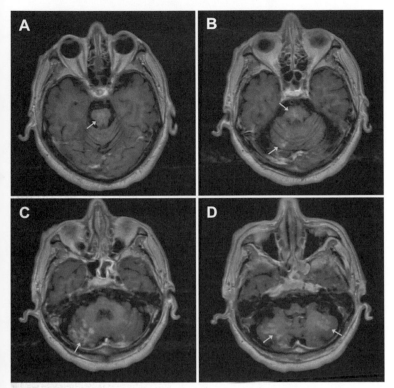

Figure 6.5 Chronic lymphocytic inflammation with pontine perivascular enhancement responsive to steroids (CLIPPERS). Axial T1 post-contrast images show punctate gadolinium-enhancing lesions involving the pons, midbrain, medulla, and cerebellum (arrows).

Chronic Lymphocytic Inflammation with Pontine Perivascular Enhancement Responsive to Steroids (CLIPPERS)

- CLIPPERS predominantly involves the pons. It typically presents with punctate, curvilinear gadolinium-enhancing pontine lesions on MRI with variable involvement of the medulla, midbrain, and spinal cord (Figure 6.5).

Myelin Oligodendrocyte Glycoprotein (MOG) Antibody Disease

- In addition to longitudinally extensive transverse myelitis (LETM), optic nerve lesions (typically bilateral) are commonly seen in MOG antibody disease (Figure 6.6).

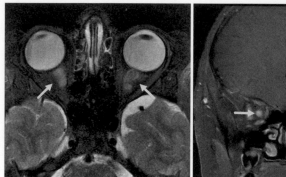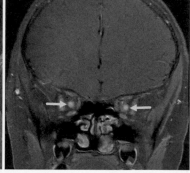

Figure 6.6 Myelin oligodendrocyte glycoprotein (MOG) antibody disease. Axial T2 fat suppression sequence (A) and coronal T1 post-contrast (B) show bilateral optic neuritis with gadolinium enhancement.

- Optic chiasm involvement is also typical (Figure 6.7).

Multiple Sclerosis

- Classic MS lesions are small but should be larger than 3 mm, ovoid, well circumscribed, and perpendicularly oriented to the lateral ventricles and the corpus callosum. They appear as hyperintense (bright) on T2/FLAIR sequencing.
- Other typical locations include juxtacortical/cortical, infratentorial, and spinal cord lesions.
- Typical MRI scans in patients with MS:
  - In clinically isolated syndrome (CIS), the MRI shows MS-like lesions disseminated in space, but no evidence of dissemination in time (no T1 black holes and no enhancing lesions) following an initial MS attack (**Figure 6.8**).
  - Confluent periventricular lesions (Figure 6.9), suggestive of high lesion burden, may develop over time when additional lesions form near each other in patients with a history of longstanding MS.
  - "Dirty" white matter (Figure 6.10) refers to areas of intermediate signal intensity between those of focal lesions and normal-appearing white matter. They are typically seen in the deep white matter.
  - Periventricular lesions (Figure 6.11), along with ventricular enlargement suggestive of brain atrophy, can be seen in some patients with longstanding MS.

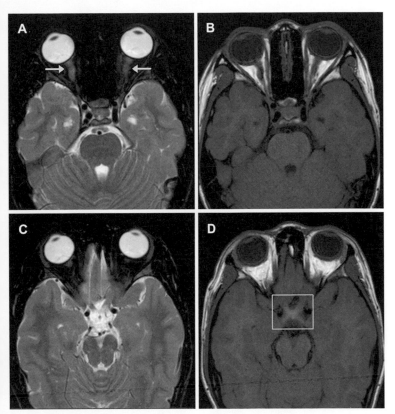

Figure 6.7 Myelin oligodendrocyte glycoprotein (MOG) antibody disease. Axial T2 fat suppression sequence (A, C) and T1 post-contrast (B) imaging show bilateral optic neuritis with enhancement of both nerves (arrows) and optic chiasm (box).

- Radiologically isolated syndrome (RIS) (Figure 6.12) is diagnosed when a brain MRI shows evidence of dissemination in space and time of MS-like lesions in a patient with no history of clinical neurologic deficits or attacks.
- Spinal cord lesions (Figure 6.13) in MS are typically small (less than 3 vertebral segments in length) and most commonly affect the posterolateral regions.
- Figure 6.14 provides a side-by-side comparison of spinal cord MRI lesions seen in MS, MOG antibody disease, and neuromyelitis optica

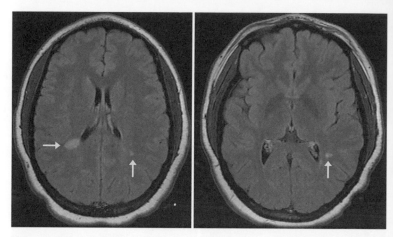

Figure 6.8 Clinically isolated syndrome (CIS). Both axial T2/FLAIR images show periventricular and white matter lesions typical of MS (arrows) meeting the criteria for dissemination in space (DIS). In a patient presenting with a first clinical event, the absence of enhancing or hypointense lesions on T1-weighted imaging (not shown) does not offer evidence of dissemination in time (DIT).

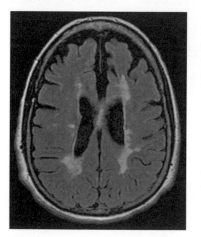

Figure 6.9 Axial T2/FLAIR image showing confluent periventricular lesions and frontal atrophy in a patient with a history of longstanding MS.

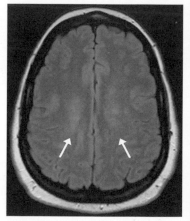

Figure 6.10 Axial T2/FLAIR image showing "dirty-appearing" white matter (arrows) in a patient with MS.

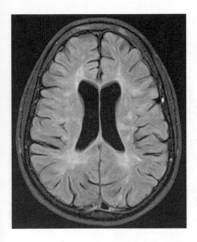

Figure 6.11 Axial T2/FLAIR image showing multiple periventricular lesions along with ventricular enlargement suggestive of brain atrophy in a patient with longstanding MS.

spectrum disorder (NMOSD). Figure 6.15 is a diagrammatic illustration of typical spinal cord lesion locations in MS and its common mimics.

- MRI scans in patients with additional findings either related or unrelated to MS:

    . Brain atrophy can occur despite the absence of high lesion volume (Figure 6.16). This could be due to degenerative changes and possible involvement of normal-appearing white matter.

    . Vascular disease may occur in addition to high periventricular lesion burden (Figure 6.17).

NMDA Receptor (NMDAR) Encephalitis

- Brain MRI may show medial temporal lobe hyperintensities, as are typical in limbic encephalitis (Figure 6.18), but is most commonly normal.

Neuromyelitis Optica Spectrum Disorder

- NMOSD lesions are typically large and edematous. Brain MRI may show optic nerve and/or brainstem lesions (Figure 6.19).
- Spinal cord lesions shown on MRI, by definition, are longitudinally extensive, spanning three or more vertebral segments (Figure 6.20).

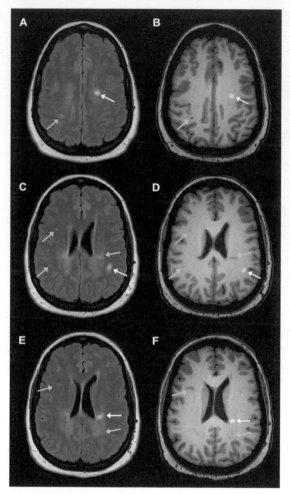

Figure 6.12
Radiographically isolated syndrome (RIS). Axial T2/FLAIR (A, C, E) and T1 post-contrast (B, D, F) images show MS-like lesions, which appear hyperintense on T2/FLAIR and hypointense on T1 (orange arrows), as well as T2/FLAIR lesions that are enhanced on T1 (white arrows), meeting the criteria for dissemination in both time and space in a patient with no history of neurologic deficits or clinical attacks.

Neurosarcoidosis

- Pachymeningeal or leptomeningeal enhancement is most common. Nonspecific T2/FLAIR hyperintensities along the base of the brain and brainstem, with or without optic nerve involvement, can also be seen (Figure 6.21).

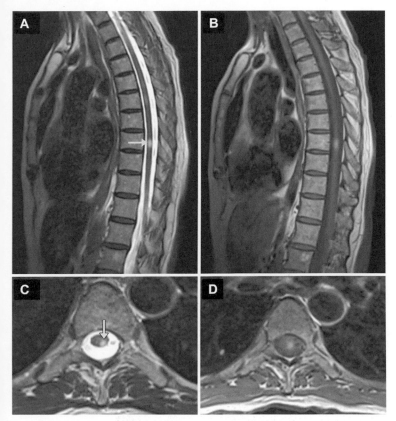

Figure 6.13 Sagittal (A) and axial (C) T1-post contrast and sagittal (B) and axial (D) T2-weighted images of the spinal cord showing an enhancing thoracic cord lesion typical of multiple sclerosis (arrows).

Progressive Multifocal Leukoencephalopathy (PML)

- Large hyperintense areas on T2/FLAIR, typically new compared to a previous scan, and most commonly without enhancement, are characteristic of PML (Figure 6.22).
- PML is a complication of prolonged use of some disease-modifying therapies for MS, such as natalizumab.

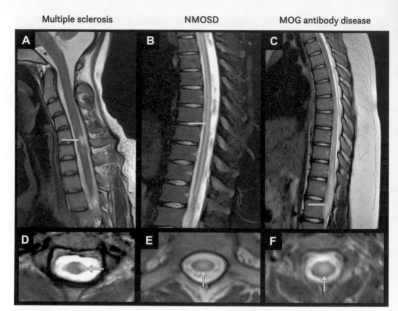

Figure 6.14 Comparison of spinal cord imaging in multiple sclerosis (A, D), neuromyelitis optica spectrum disorder [NMOSD] (B, E), and myelin oligodendrocyte glycoprotein (MOG) antibody disease (C, F). MS lesions are short (less than 3 vertebral segments in length) (A) and affect the peripheral cord (D), whereas those of NMOSD (B) and MOG antibody disease (C) are typically longitudinally extensive (greater than 3 vertebral segments in length) and more commonly affect the central cord (E, F).

Sjögren Syndrome

- Optic neuritis may be present in some cases. Spinal cord involvement, if present, is usually longitudinally extensive, spanning more than three vertebral segments. Honeycomb appearance of the parotid gland and/or lacrimal gland or duct enhancement may be seen (Figure 6.23).

Weston–Hurst Syndrome

- Also known as acute hemorrhagic leukoencephalitis, Weston–Hurst syndrome is a rare variant of ADEM that is usually fatal.

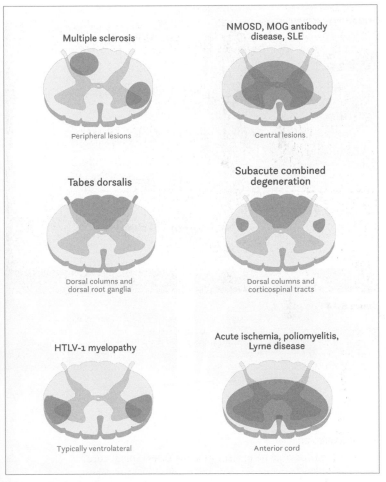

Figure 6.15 Typical location of lesions in multiple sclerosis and its mimics. Abbreviations: MOG, myelin oligodendrocyte glycoprotein; NMOSD, neuromyelitis optica spectrum disorder, SLE, systemic lupus erythematous.

- MRI typically shows large demyelinating lesions with associated hemorrhages and an extensive mass effect with surrounding edema (Figure 6.24).
- Susceptibility-weighted images (SWI) are an important sequence that allows for differentiation of Weston–Hurst syndrome from ADEM. Hemorrhagic areas appear dark on SWI.

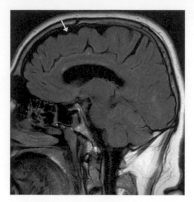

Figure 6.16 Frontoparietal brain atrophy in a patient with MS in the absence of high lesion burden (arrow).

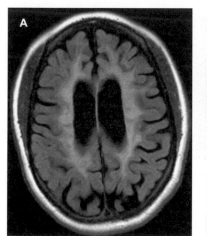
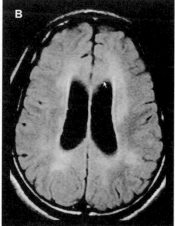

Figure 6.17 (A) Axial T2/FLAIR image showing high periventricular lesion burden in a patient with MS in addition to vascular ischemic changes (based on history) and ventricular enlargement due to brain atrophy. (B) Axial T2/FLAIR image showing microvascular changes in a patient without MS.

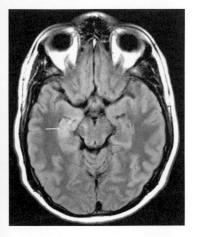

Figure 6.18 NMDA receptor encephalitis. T2/FLAIR hyperintense signal involving the mesial temporal lobe.

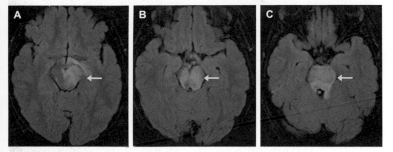

Figure 6.19 Neuromyelitis optica spectrum disorder (NMOSD). Axial T2/FLAIR images showing a hyperintense signal involving the midbrain (A, B) and pons with extension into the cerebellum (C).

Hereditary/Genetic Diseases
Cerebral Autosomal Dominant Arteriopathy with Subcortical Infarcts and Leukoencephalopathy (CADASIL)

- MRI typically shows diffuse white matter changes with anterior temporal and external capsule involvement (Figure 6.25).

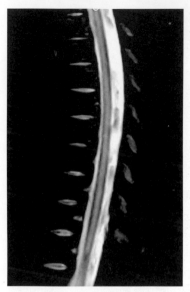

Figure 6.20 Neuromyelitis optica spectrum disorder (NMOSD). Sagittal T2 spinal cord imaging showing a typical longitudinally extensive (more than three vertebral segments) NMOSD lesion (arrow).

Leukodystrophies

- **Metachromatic leukodystrophy (MLD)**

  - MLD is the most common hereditary leukodystrophy. Its characteristic imaging features include diffuse dysmyelination with periventricular perivenular sparing, resulting in a "tigroid" pattern of the white matter on MRI (Figure 6.26).

Mitochondrial Disease

- **Leigh syndrome**

  - Leigh syndrome is one of many mitochondrial disorders resulting from genetic mutations in both nuclear and mitochondrial DNA. Common MRI features include bihemispheric T2/FLAIR hyperintense signal changes, typically involving white and gray matter and the brainstem (Figure 6.27).

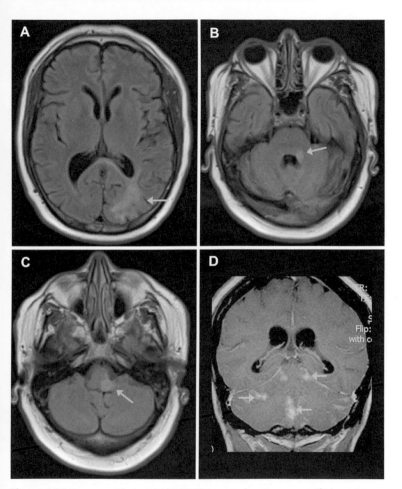

Figure 6.21 Neurosarcoidosis. Axial T2/FLAIR images showing nonspecific hyperintense white matter lesions in the occipital lobe (A) and brainstem (B, C). Panel D shows a T1 post-contrast image of a different patient with neurosarcoidosis and predominantly cerebellar involvement (arrows).

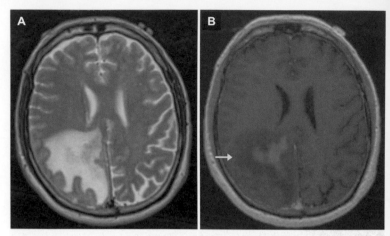

Figure 6.22 Progressive multifocal leukoencephalopathy (PML). Axial T2 (A) and T1 post-contrast (B) images show a large T2 hyperintense right hemispheric lesion with surrounding edema and no gadolinium enhancement (arrows).

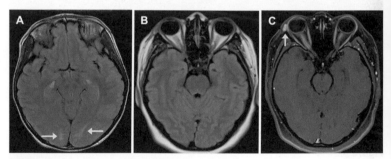

Figure 6.23 Sjögren syndrome. Axial T2/FLAIR (A, B) and T1 post-contrast (C) images show nonspecific T2 hyperintensities in the occipital white matter bilaterally (A, arrows), as well as right lacrimal gland enhancement (C, arrow).

Infectious Diseases
Cryptococcal Meningitis

- Patients with cryptococcal meningitis usually present with meningitis or meningoencephalitis. Radiographic features include hydrocephalus, leptomeningeal enhancement, T2/FLAIR hyperintensities, and nodular enhancement of parenchymal lesions (Figure 6.28).

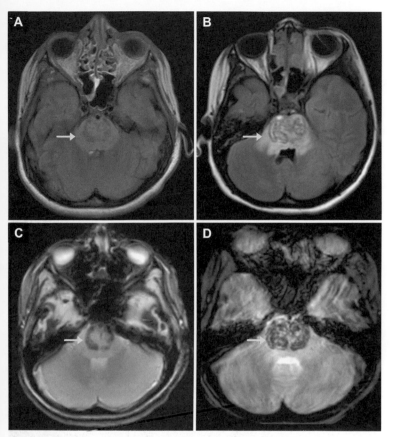

Figure 6.24 Weston–Hurst syndrome (acute hemorrhagic leukoencephalitis). Axial T2/FLAIR (A, B) and susceptibility-weighted imaging (SWI) images (C, D) show extensive punctate areas of hemorrhage involving the brainstem (arrows).

Human T-Lymphotropic Virus Type 1 (HTLV-1)

- HTLV-1 infection is also known as tropical spastic paraparesis and HTLV-1 associated myelopathy. The most common presentation is a slowly progressive chronic spastic paraparesis with bowel and bladder dysfunction and lower limb sensory disturbance.
- The most common MRI feature is cord atrophy and increased signals in the lateral columns, mostly involving the white matter (Figure 6.29).

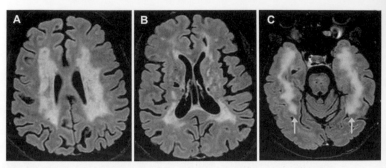

Figure 6.25 Cerebral autosomal dominant arteriopathy with subcortical infarcts and leukoencephalopathy.(CADASIL). Axial T2/FLAIR images show diffuse white matter changes in both hemispheres with anterior temporal involvement (C, arrows).

Lyme Disease (Neuroborreliosis)

- *Borrelia burgdorferi* infections may involve the CNS in some cases. Typical associated symptoms include erythema migrans and other systemic symptoms.
- Brain MRI in patients with Lyme disease is typically normal. When present, findings may include subcortical areas of T2 hyperintensity and meningeal enhancement (Figure 6.30).

Tabes Dorsalis (Neurosyphilis)

- MRI findings for patients with neurosyphilis may include leptomeningeal enhancement, cerebral atrophy, or T2-weighted hyperintensities in the dorsal columns of the spinal cord (Figure 6.31).

Metabolic Diseases
Vitamin B$_{12}$ Deficiency (Subacute Combined Degeneration)

- MRI findings in case of vitamin B$_{12}$ deficiency typically include symmetric bilateral increased T2 signals within the dorsal columns, most commonly involving the upper thoracic region (Figure 6.32).

Neoplastic Disease
Lymphoma

- Typical lymphoma lesions may show homogeneous enhancement on T1 sequencing, whereas peripheral ring lesion enhancement may be seen in immunocompromised patients (Figure 6.33).

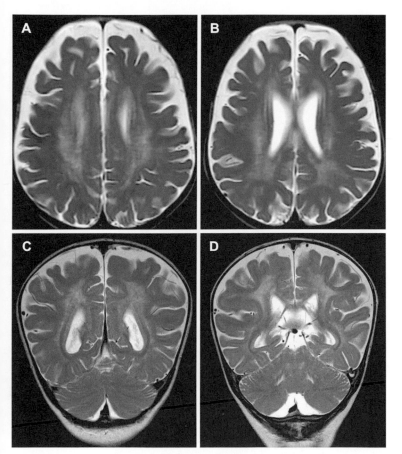

Figure 6.26 Metachromatic leukodystrophy (MLD). Axial (A, B) and coronal (C, D) T2-weighted scans show the typical "tigroid" pattern of white matter dysmyelination.

Medulloblastoma

- Medulloblastomas are among the most common malignant tumors of childhood. They typically lead to a rapid onset of neurologic deficits.

- MRI may show lesions with areas of T2/FLAIR hyperintensity due to necrosis and cyst formation with surrounding edema. Most lesions are enhanced heterogeneously with contrast.

- These tumors most often involve the cerebellum (Figure 6.34).

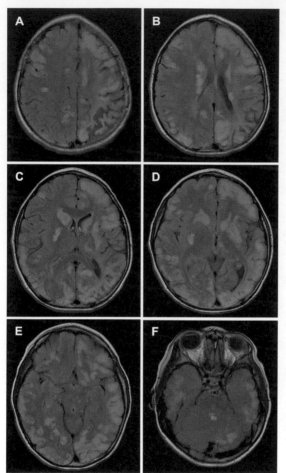

Figure 6.27 Leigh syndrome. Axial T2/FLAIR scans show bihemispheric areas of hyperintense signal changes involving both white and gray matter, as well as the brainstem.

Meningioma

- Most meningiomas are found incidentally and are asymptomatic. Often, they may result in headaches or a variety of other symptoms, including motor deficits or changes in mental status.
- These tumors are most commonly supratentorial in location. They may appear as iso-intense to hyperintense masses with homogeneous enhancement on T1-weighted sequencing (Figure 6.35).

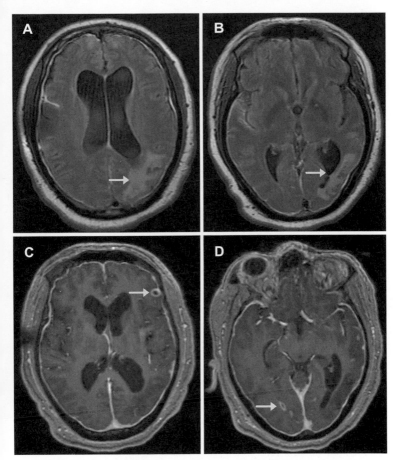

Figure 6.28 Cryptococcal meningitis. Axial T2/FLAIR (A, B) and T1 post-contrast (C, D) scans show a T2/FLAIR hyperintense area in the left temporo-occipital lobe (A, B; arrows), as well as nodular enhancement of parenchymal lesions (C, D; arrows). Diffuse leptomeningeal enhancement is also seen throughout.

Glioblastoma Multiforme

- Glioblastomas are typically large tumors with thick, irregular enhancing margins and a central necrotic core. They may be surrounded by vasogenic edema.
- Enhancement on MRI is variable, but almost always present in a ring configuration (Figure 6.36).

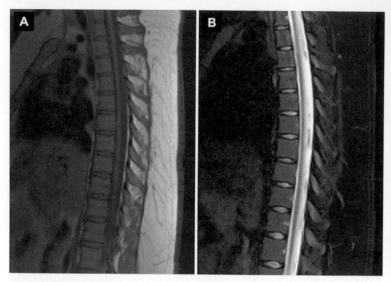

Figure 6.29 HTLV-1 myelopathy. Sagittal T1 post-contrast (A) and T2 (B) scans show atrophy of the spinal cord.

Trauma
Vertebral Fracture

- Different types of vertebral fractures may occur. Fractured vertebral bodies are commonly seen after blunt trauma and are evident on MRI (Figure 6.37).

Vascular Disease
Antiphospholipid Syndrome

- Thoracic spinal cord involvement is common with antiphospholipid syndrome. When present, brain MRI findings are typically consistent with ischemic stroke/thrombotic events (Figure 6.38).

Arteriovenous Malformation

- Arteriovenous malformation lesions are characterized by an abnormal leash of vessels that allow for arteriovenous shunting. Typical radiographic features include signal voids from high-velocity flow, with increased T2 signals from cytotoxic edema or encephalomalacia/myelomalacia (Figure 6.39).

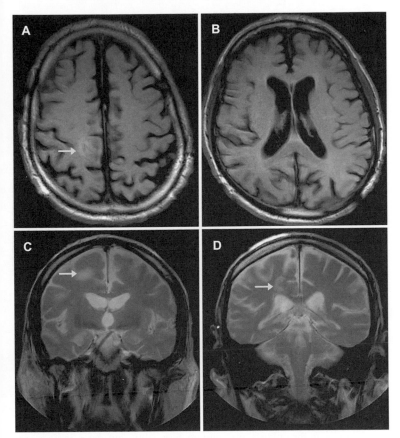

Figure 6.30 Contrast scans showing a cerebellar mass with heterogeneous enhancement, including nonspecific areas of T2 hyperintensity (C, D; arrows) and faint enhancement of one of the lesions in the right hemisphere (A, arrow), in a patient with active Lyme disease.

Behçet Disease

- Behçet disease is a multisystemic and chronic inflammatory vasculitis of unknown etiology.
- MRI findings can be abnormal in as many as two-thirds of patients. They may show focal/multifocal lesions (brainstem lesions are most common),

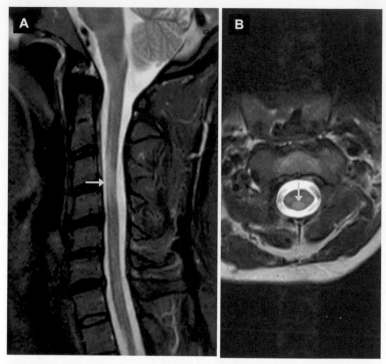

Figure 6.31 Tabes dorsalis (neurosyphilis). Sagittal T1 post-contrast (A) and axial T2 (B) scans show a spinal cord lesion (A, arrow) with involvement of the posterior columns (B, arrow).

cerebral vein thrombosis, or meningoencephalitis, but these findings are nonspecific (Figure 6.40).

Hemorrhagic Stroke

- T1-weighted sequencing with contrast may help reveal leakage across the blood–brain barrier. Increased and/or decreased T1 and T2/FLAIR signal changes over time can help estimate the age of a hemorrhagic stroke.
- Hemorrhagic areas will appear dark on susceptibility-weighted imaging (Figure 6.41).
- Hemorrhagic strokes are more typically identified via computed tomography (CT) scan in the acute setting.

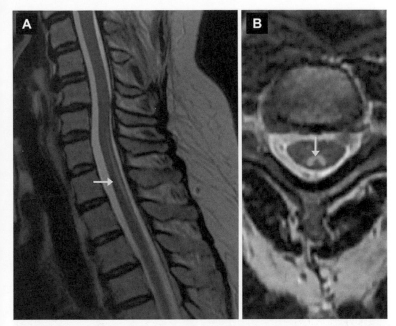

Figure 6.32 Subacute combined degeneration (vitamin B$_{12}$ deficiency). Sagittal (A) and axial (B) T2 scans show an area of T2 hyperintense signal within the spinal cord, with involvement of the dorsal columns (arrows).

Ischemic Stroke

- When ischemic stroke is suspected, CT, CT angiography (CTA), and CT perfusion are commonly used diagnostic tools in the acute setting.
- MRI is more time consuming than CT and, therefore, less commonly used as a diagnostic tool for acute strokes.
- T2/FLAIR hyperintensities are often seen in ischemic areas, and T1 contrast enhancement may be seen days later. However, diffusion-weighted imaging (DWI) and apparent diffusion coefficient (ADC) sequencing are most commonly used in the acute setting to identify ischemic strokes. Such areas appear bright on DWI and dark on ADC (Figure 6.42).

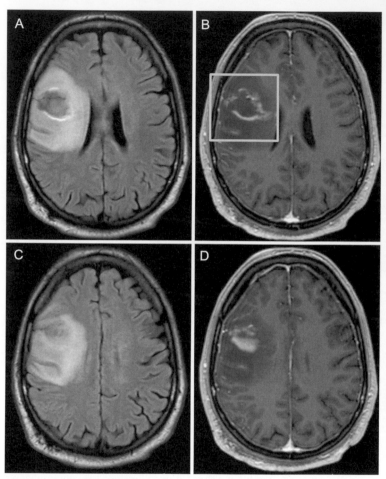

Figure 6.33 Lymphoma. Axial T2/FLAIR (A, C) and T1 post-contrast (B, D) images show a large mass-like lesion in the right hemisphere with surrounding edema and a rim of gadolinium enhancement (box).

Susac Syndrome

- Susac syndrome is characterized by the triad of acute to subacute encephalopathy, bilateral sensorineural hearing loss, and branch retinal artery occlusions.

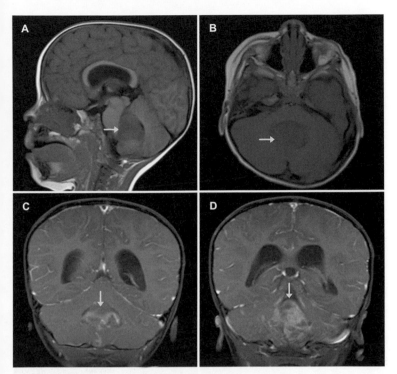

Figure 6.34 Medulloblastoma. Sagittal (A) and axial (B) T1-weighted and coronal (C, D) T1 post-contrast scans show a cerebellar mass with heterogeneous enhancement.

- Characteristic MRI features include rounded T2 hyperintense "snowball" lesions with involvement of the corpus callosum. Leptomeningeal and gray matter enhancement may also be present (Figure 6.43).

Vasculitis

- Vasculitis refers to generalized inflammation of vessels and can involve almost any organ system. It has a number of possible etiologies.
- CNS vasculitis may occur as a result of autoimmune diseases including systemic lupus erythematosus, granulomatosis with polyangiitis,

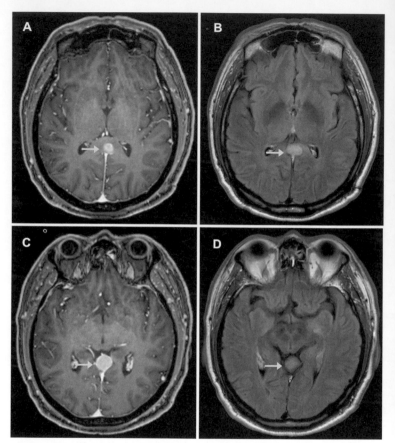

Figure 6.35 Meningioma. Axial T1 post-contrast (A, C) and T2/FLAIR (B, D) scans show a T2/FLAIR hyperintense mass with homogeneous gadolinium enhancement (arrows).

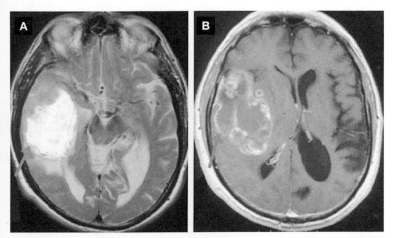

Figure 6.36 Axial T2 (A) and T1 post-contrast (B) images show glioblastoma multiforme.

rheumatoid arthritis, Behçet syndrome, and other conditions such as inflammatory arteritis and infectious diseases.
- Angiography shows focal or multifocal segmental narrowing of small and medium-sized blood vessels. In some cases, occlusions may be present.
- MRI findings may be consistent with infarctions. They are usually bilateral and show different vascular territories in various stages of healing (Figure 6.44).

Conclusion

MRI features can help differentiate MS from alternative diagnoses. However, it is important to recognize that MS may coexist with some of these disorders. Incorporating the characteristic imaging features for each condition should help improve diagnostic accuracy.

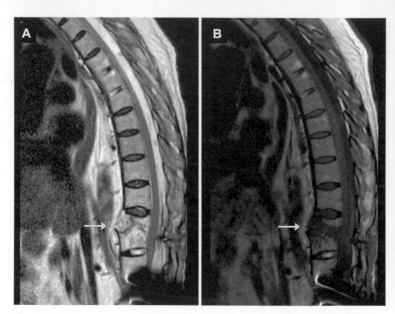

Figure 6.37 Thoracic vertebral body fracture. Sagittal T1-weighted (A) and T2-weighted (B) images show a hyperextension injury at T12, with a transversely oriented fracture disrupting the anterior longitudinal ligament (arrows).

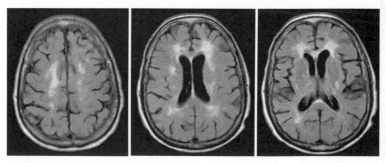

Figure 6.38 Antiphospholipid syndrome. Axial T2/FLAIR images show multiple confluent periventricular and subcortical lesions in a female patient with a history of multiple miscarriages.

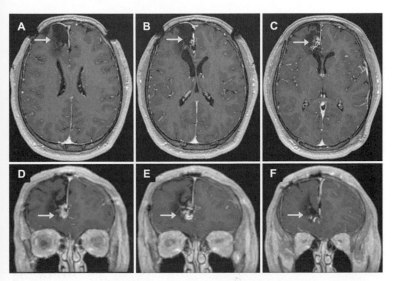

Figure 6.39 Arteriovenous malformation (AVM). Axial (A–C) and coronal (D–F) T1 post-contrast scans show an abnormal leash of blood vessels with gadolinium enhancement, surrounding edema, and signal flow voids (arrows).

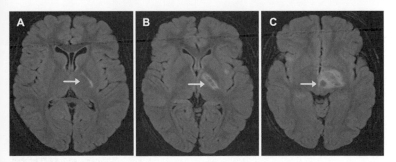

Figure 6.40 Behçet disease. Axial T2/FLAIR scans show nonspecific hyperintense signal changes involving the basal ganglia and brainstem (arrows).

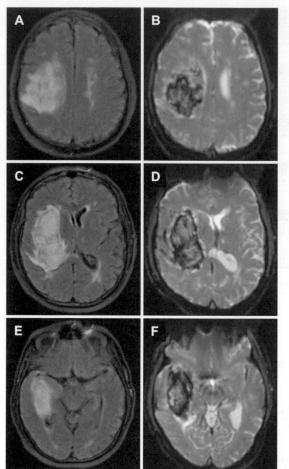

Figure 6.41
Hemorrhagic stroke. Axial T2/FLAIR (A, C, E) and susceptibility-weighted imaging (SWI) (B, D, F) scans show areas of T2/FLAIR hyperintensity, with SWI correlates (dark) representing areas of parenchymal hemorrhage.

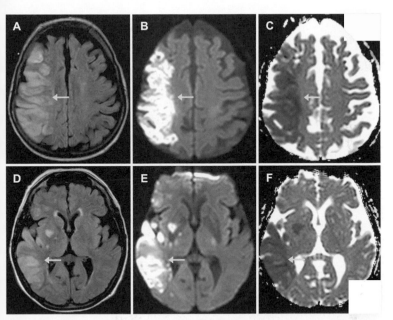

Figure 6.42 Ischemic stroke. These axial T2/FLAIR (A, D), diffusion-weighted imaging (DWI) (B, E), and apparent diffusion coefficient (ADC) (C, F) scans are consistent with a right middle cerebral artery (MCA) stroke. Ischemic areas appear hyperintense on T2/LAIR, less bright on DWI, and dark on ADC (arrows).

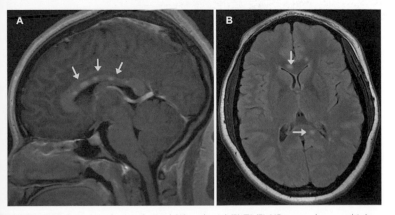

Figure 6.43 Susac syndrome. Sagittal (A) and axial (B) T2/FLAIR scans show multiple round lesions within the corpus callosum.

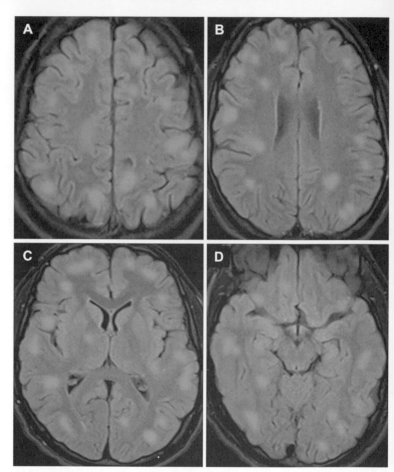

Figure 6.44 Vasculitis. Axial T2/FLAIR scans show multiple areas of high signal intensity, mostly located near the white–gray matter junction.

CLINICAL PEARLS

- MRI findings are the best surrogate marker of MS activity and disease progression.
- Patient positioning, selection of MRI sequences, administration of contrast, and magnet strength can all affect lesion detection.
- Numerous clinical and radiographic mimics of MS exist, making the diagnosis challenging.
- The McDonald diagnostic criteria for MS emphasize that there must be no "better explanation" for clinical findings than MS.
- This chapter illustrated a series of radiologic MS mimics, highlighting features that should alert the clinician to consider a wider differential diagnosis.

References

1. Ropele S, De Graaf W, Khalil M, et al. MRI assessment of iron deposition in multiple sclerosis. *J Magn Reson Imaging*. 2011;34(1):13–21. doi:10.1002/jmri.22590

2. McMahon KL, Cowin G, Galloway G. Magnetic resonance imaging: the underlying principles. *J Orthop Sport Phys Ther*. 2011;41(11):806–19. doi:10.2519/jospt.2011.3576

3. Ge Y. Multiple sclerosis: the role of MR imaging. *Am J Neuroradiol*. 2006;27 (6):1165–76. doi:27/6/1165 [pii]

4. Sands MJ, Levitin A. Basics of magnetic resonance imaging. *Semin Vasc Surg*. 2004;17(2):66–82. doi:10.1053/j.semvascsurg.2004.03.011

5. Klawiter EC. Current and new directions in MRI in multiple sclerosis. *Continuum (Minneap Minn)*. 2013:1058–73.

6. Sahraian MA, Eshaghi A. Role of MRI in diagnosis and treatment of multiple sclerosis. *Clin Neurol Neurosurg*. 2010;112(7):609–15. doi:10.1016/j.clineuro.2010.03.022

7. Pretorius PM, Quaghebeur G. The role of MRI in the diagnosis of MS. *Clin Radiol*. 2003;58(6):434–48. doi:10.1016/S0009-9260(03)00089-8

8. Hemond CC, Bakshi R. Magnetic resonance imaging in multiple sclerosis. *Cold Spring Harb Perspect Med*. 2018:a028969. doi:10.1101/cshperspect.a028969

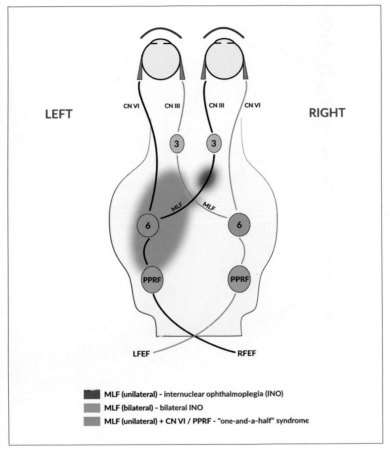

LEFT   RIGHT

CN VI   CN III   CN III   CN VI

3   3

MLF   MLF

6   6

PPRF   PPRF

LFEF   RFEF

■ **MLF (unilateral) - internuclear ophthalmoplegia (INO)**
■ **MLF (bilateral) - bilateral INO**
■ **MLF (unilateral) + CN VI / PPRF - "one-and-a-half" syndrome**

Figure 1.2 Internuclear ophthalmoplegia and other brainstem disorders of gaze. Abbreviations: CN, cranial nerve; LFEF, left frontal eye field; MLF; medial longitudinal fasciculus; PPRF, parapontine reticular formation; RFEF, right frontal eye field. (A black and white version of this figure will appear in some formats.)

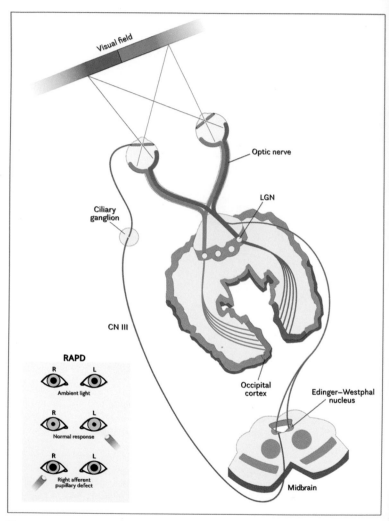

Figure 2.4 Pupillary reflex pathway. A relative afferent pupillary defect (RAPD) can result from inflammatory damage to the optic nerve. A reduced pupillary response to light is seen in which the patient's pupil appears to dilate when a light is shined onto the affected eye. (A black and white version of this figure will appear in some formats.)

A

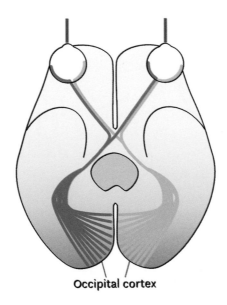

Occipital cortex

B

Normal

P100

Abnormal

P100

50 msec

Figure 4.8 Visual evoked potentials (VEPs). (A) A visual stimulus, such as an alternating checkerboard pattern on a computer screen, is given to a patient. The time it takes for the stimulus to reach the occipital cortex (P100) is measured. A delay in electrical signal conduction is suggestive of current (or prior) demyelination of the optic nerve. (A black and white version of this figure will appear in some formats.)

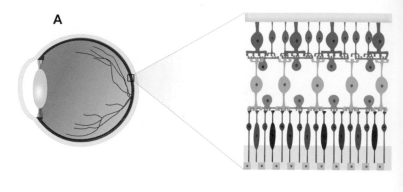

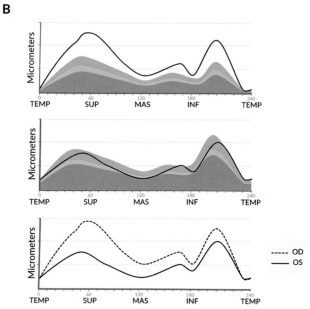

Figure 4.9 Optical coherence tomography (OCT) obtains high-resolution images of the retina (A). Axonal thickness is then measured (B). A decrease in retinal thickness may be suggestive of prior demyelination of the optic nerve. (A black and white version of this figure will appear in some formats.)

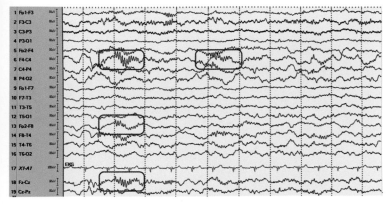

Figure 5.4 Electroencephalogram (EEG) showing a "delta brush" pattern consisting of diffuse delta slowing with superimposed high-frequency activity (red boxes) in a patient with NMDAR encephalitis. (A black and white version of this figure will appear in some formats.)

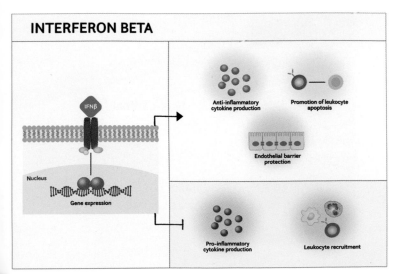

Figure 7.2 Mechanism of action of interferons. (A black and white version of this figure will appear in some formats.)

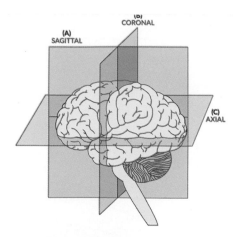

Figure 6.1 Typical locations of multiple sclerosis lesions in the sagittal (A), coronal (B), and axial (C) planes. (A black and white version of this figure will appear in some formats.)

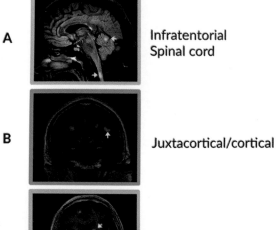

A   Infratentorial
Spinal cord

B   Juxtacortical/cortical

C   Periventricular

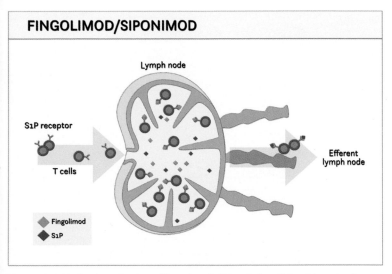

Figure 7.6 Mechanism of action of fingolimod. Abbreviation: S1P, sphingosine-1-phosphate. (A black and white version of this figure will appear in some formats.)

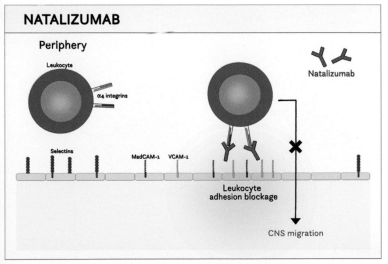

Figure 7.8 Mechanism of action of natalizumab. (A black and white version of this figure will appear in some formats.)

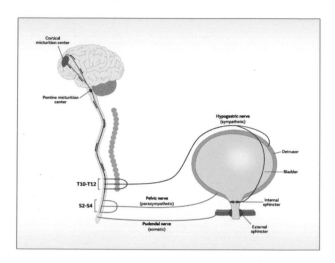

Figure 9.1 Bladder innervation. The bladder receives motor input from both sympathetic (hypogastric nerve) and parasympathetic (pelvic nerve) sources. Sensation from the bladder is transmitted to the micturition center in the brain, which then allows for voluntary control of the external sphincter via the pudendal nerve. Dyssynergia between any of these connections can lead to urinary incontinence. The hypogastric nerve acts on the internal sphincter via alpha-1 receptors. The pudendal nerve acts on the external sphincter via nicotinic acetylcholine receptors. (A black and white version of this figure will appear in some formats.)

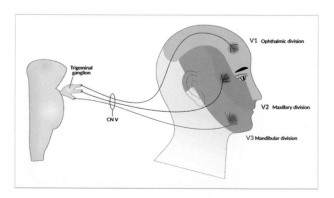

Figure 9.2 Trigeminal neuralgia pathophysiology. The trigeminal nerve (CN V) carries sensory information from the face to the brain. Inflammatory lesions may result in severe pain along any of its branches (V1, V2, V3). (A black and white version of this figure will appear in some formats.)

Disease-Modifying Therapies

Carlos A. Pérez, MD

Chapter 7

With the ongoing expansion of the therapeutic armamentarium, treatment strategies for multiple sclerosis (MS) have undergone profound changes in the last few years. Several treatment options are available at this time, and the effects of these drugs appear to be greater when treatment is initiated early, soon after the onset of symptoms. This chapter reviews currently used disease-modifying agents (Figure 7.1) in addition to several promising therapies in various phases of development.

Immunomodulatory Agents

Injectable Therapies

Self-injectable (intramuscular and subcutaneous) therapies emerged as the first disease-modifying therapy (DMT) for MS.[1-3]

Interferons (Avonex, Betaseron, Extavia, Plegridy, Rebif)

- Interferons are the most widely used first-line DMT in MS. Their exact mechanism of action is unknown but may include stabilization of the

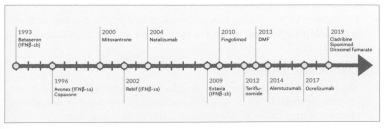

Figure 7.1 Timeline of FDA approval for currently available disease-modifying therapies (DMTs).

INTERFERON BETA

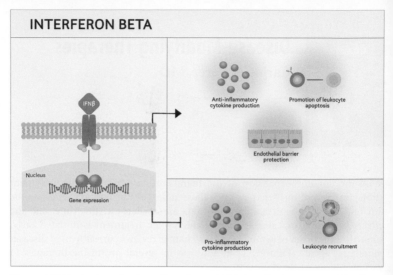

Figure 7.2 Mechanism of action of interferons. (A black and white version of this figure will appear in some formats. For the colour version, please refer to the plate section.)

blood–brain barrier and promotion of a shift from a pro-inflammatory to an anti-inflammatory milieu[1] (Figure 7.2).

- These agents have been shown to reduce relapse rates and new activity shown on magnetic resonance imaging (MRI), as well as delay disability progression[3] as measured by the Expanded Disability Status Scale (EDSS; Appendix 1).
- Interferons have a well-known and favorable safety profile with established long-term efficacy. Possible side effects may include flu-like symptoms, depression, hepatotoxicity, lymphopenia, and injection-site reactions including necrosis.[4]
- The efficacy of interferons can be compromised by the development of neutralizing antibodies, which are more common with high-frequency formulations.[4]

Glatiramer Acetate (Copaxone)

- Glatiramer acetate is a synthetic protein that simulates the myelin basic protein. Its mechanism of action is unclear, but this agent is thought to promote upregulation of T-regulatory cells, inducing an anti-inflammatory milieu (Figure 7.3).
- The pivotal studies showed efficacy in reducing relapse rates and MRI activity. Glatiramer acetate has no effect on disability progression.[3]

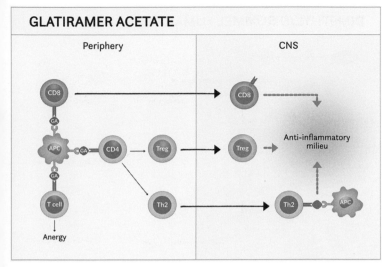

Figure 7.3 Mechanism of action of glatiramer acetate. Abbreviations: APC, antigen-presenting cell; GA, glatiramer acetate.

- It is known to have an excellent long-term profile. Side effects include injection-site reactions. Serious adverse effects are uncommon.[5]

Daclizumab (Zinbryta)

- Daclizumab was withdrawn from the market worldwide on March 2, 2018, due to reports of severe adverse effects, including hepatotoxicity, encephalitis, and meningoencephalitis.[3]
- This humanized monoclonal antibody binds to the alpha chain component of the interleukin-2 receptor and was shown to be effective in reducing relapse rates and disability.[6]

Oral Therapies

The oral medications are relatively new additions to the therapeutic armamentarium for MS and trade the convenience of an oral formulation for the long-term safety profile of the injectable medications.

Dimethyl Fumarate (Tecfidera)

- Dimethyl fumarate may exert its anti-inflammatory and neuroprotective/antioxidant effects based on its action on the nuclear factor-kappa

DIMETHYL/DIROXIMEL FUMARATE

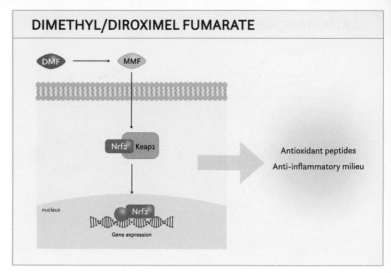

Figure 7.4 Mechanism of action of dimethyl fumarate (and diroximel fumarate). Abbreviations: DMF, dimethyl fumarate; MMF, monomethyl fumarate.

B (NF-κB) and nuclear factor erythroid 2–related factor 2 (Nrf-2) pathways, respectively[6,7] (Figure 7.4).
- It has been shown to reduce relapse rates and new MRI activity.[3]
- Side effects include flushing (which may improve with use of daily aspirin), gastrointestinal upset (nausea, diarrhea, abdominal pain), and lymphopenia. Rare cases of progressive multifocal leukoencephalopathy (PML) have been reported.[6]

Teriflunomide (Aubagio)
- Teriflunomide is an inhibitor of dihydroorotate, an enzyme involved in pyrimidine synthesis. It acts by reducing the proliferation of pro-inflammatory lymphocytes[6] (Figure 7.5).
- Clinical studies have shown efficacy in reducing relapse rates, MRI activity, and disability progression.[3]
- Common safety concerns include hepatotoxicity and infection.[6]
- Teriflunomide is classified in FDA pregnancy Category X. This agent is detectable in seminal fluid, so sexually active males who take this medication should consider contraceptive techniques as well.[8,9]

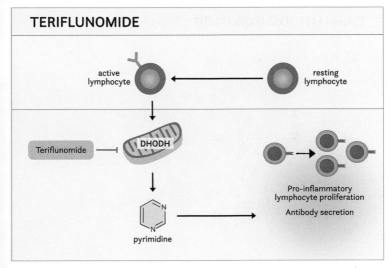

Figure 7.5 Mechanism of action of teriflunomide. Abbreviation: DHODH, dihydroorotate dehydrogenase.

Fingolimod (Gilenya)

- Fingolimod is a sphingosine 1-phosphate receptor modulator that is thought to act by retaining lymphocytes (including autoreactive lymphocytes) in the lymph nodes[1,10] (Figure 7.6).
- Clinical trials have shown positive data for reducing relapses, MRI activity, and rate of brain atrophy.[3] The risk of herpetic infections (including varicella) is higher with fingolimod, so ensuring immunity against the varicella virus prior to initiating fingolimod is prudent.[2]
- Potential side effects include first-dose cardiac bradyarrhythmia, macular edema, and hepatotoxicity.[9]

Siponimod (Mayzent)

- Like fingolimod, siponimod is a sphingosine 1-phosphate receptor modulator that is thought to act by retaining lymphocytes (including autoreactive lymphocytes) in the lymph nodes[1,10] (Figure 7.6).
- According to the most recent Phase III clinical trial data, siponimod may reduce disease activity and has a modest effect on the gradual accrual of disability. It was approved by the Food and Drug Administration (FDA) for treatment of secondary progressive multiple sclerosis.[11]

FINGOLIMOD/SIPONIMOD

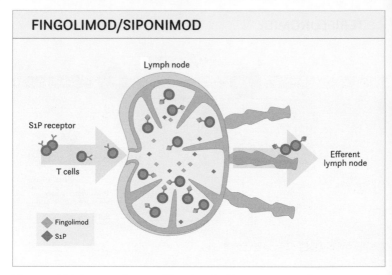

Figure 7.6 Mechanism of action of fingolimod. Abbreviation: S1P, sphingosine-1-phosphate. (A black and white version of this figure will appear in some formats. For the colour version, please refer to the plate section.)

- Potential side effects include headache, high blood pressure, and liver function test abnormalities. Siponimod has fewer cardiac side effects than fingolimod.

Cladribine (Mavenclad)

- Cladribine is a purine analog that targets lymphocytes and selectively suppresses the immune system. It acts by mimicking the nucleoside adenosine and triggers apoptosis of lymphocytes (Figure 7.7).
- It is currently approved for the treatment of relapsing-remitting MS and active secondary progressive MS.
- Clinical studies have shown reductions of annual relapse rates and disability progression.[12]
- This agent is contraindicated in patients who have cancer or human immunodeficiency virus (HIV) infection, and in those who are pregnant or breastfeeding.
- Associated risks include increased risk of cancer and birth defects.

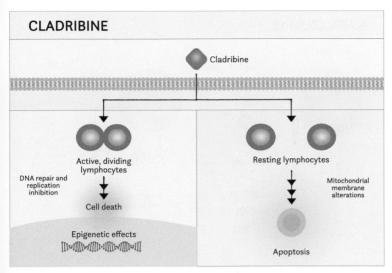

Figure 7.7 Mechanism of action of cladribine.

- Other side effects include lymphopenia, anemia, infections, headache, sore throat, flu-like illness, and nausea.

Infusion Therapies

The intravenous (IV) therapies favor efficacy at the expense of safety, so they arc less likely to be used in early MS.

Natalizumab (Tysabri)

- Natalizumab is a synthetic monoclonal antibody that selectively inhibits VLA-4 ($\alpha 4\beta 1$) integrins, preventing leukocyte migration across the blood–brain barrier[1,13] (Figure 7.8).
- It has been shown to reduce relapse rates and disability progression, and also has a profound effect on MRI activity.[3]
- Common side effects are usually mild and include mild infusion reactions (e.g., headache, fever). If a hypersensitivity reaction develops (e.g., urticaria, dermatitis, bronchospasm), discontinuation is recommended due to the risk of anaphylaxis with subsequent infusions.[1,7]

NATALIZUMAB

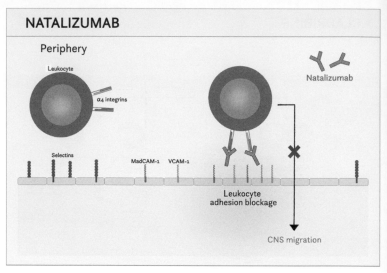

Figure 7.8 Mechanism of action of natalizumab. (A black and white version of this figure will appear in some formats. For the colour version, please refer to the plate section.)

- Cessation of natalizumab treatment in the absence of bridge therapy (i.e., steroids) or the introduction of a fast-acting DMT has been associated with disease rebound after three to four months.[14]
- Natalizumab has been associated with the activation of latent JC virus infection known to cause PML. The risk can be further stratified based on the presence of serum JC virus antibody, length of treatment, and prior use of immunosuppressive therapies.[15]
- Rarely, efficacy of the agent may be compromised by the development of neutralizing antibodies.[3]

Alemtuzumab (Lemtrada)

- Alemtuzumab is a humanized monoclonal antibody directed at CD52, a protein on the surface of lymphocytes, which results in B- and T-cell lysis and activation of T cells by an unclear mechanism[1,2] (Figure 7.9).
- Clinical studies have shown a reduction of relapse rates and MRI activity.[3]
- Mild infusion reactions can occur. Alemtuzumab is also known to cause profound and long-lasting alterations in lymphocyte counts (up to two years or more) and carries an almost 30% chance of secondary

ALEMTUZUMAB

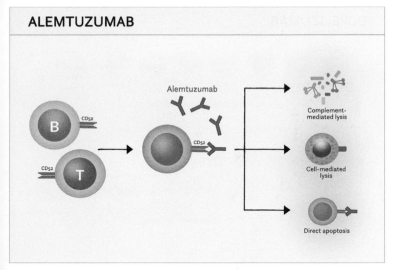

Figure 7.9 Mechanism of action of alemtuzumab.

autoimmunity (mostly thyroid), with potential long-term risk of malignancy.[6]

Ocrelizumab (Ocrevus)

- Ocrelizumab is a humanized monoclonal antibody that targets CD20 on B cells through mechanisms that induce antibody-dependent cell-mediated cytotoxicity and/or the induction of apoptosis[10] (Figure 7.10).
- Clinical studies have shown it produces a reduction of relapse rates, MRI activity, and disability progression.[3]
- This agent is contraindicated in patients with active hepatitis B virus infection, so patients must be screened for hepatitis B virus before starting ocrelizumab. In addition, live-attenuated and live vaccines are not recommended during ocrelizumab treatment or after discontinuation until B-cell repletion occurs.[7,10]

Other Therapies
Azathioprine (Imuran)

- Azathioprine is a derivative of mercaptopurine that blocks purine synthesis and halts replication, preventing the proliferation of T and B- ymphocytes[16] (Figure 7.11).

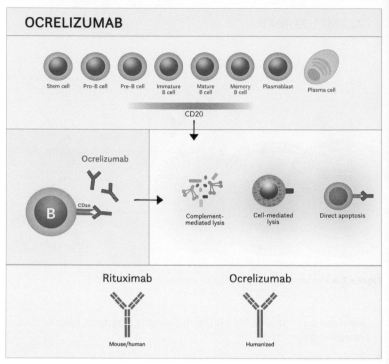

Figure 7.10 Mechanism of action of ocrelizumab (and rituximab).

- Pivotal studies showed a decrease in relapse rates and disease progression in patients with MS.[3]
- Possible side effects include severe nausea, anemia or leukopenia, and hepatotoxicity.[16]
- Chronic immunosuppression (lasting more than five years) with this agent increases the risk of malignancy.[3]

Cyclophosphamide (Cytoxan)

- Cyclophosphamide is an immunosuppressant that works by binding to cell DNA and interfering with division and replication of T and B lymphocytes[17] (Figure 7.12).
- Several clinical trials demonstrated it produces reduction of relapses and MRI activity in patients with MS.[3]

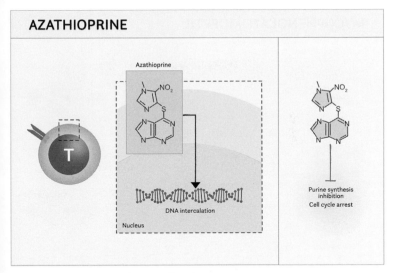

Figure 7.11 Mechanism of action of azathioprine.

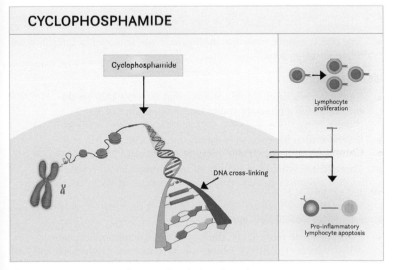

Figure 7.12 Mechanism of action of cyclophosphamide.

MYCOPHENOLATE MOFETIL

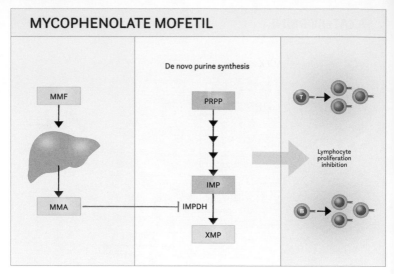

Figure 7.13 Mechanism of action of mycophenolate mofetil. Abbreviations: IMP, inosine monophosphate; IMPDH, inosine monophosphate dehydrogenase; MMA, mycophenolic acid; MMF, mycophenolate mofetil; XMP, xanthine monophosphate.

- Side effects include nausea, vomiting, hair loss, leukopenia, infertility, and hemorrhagic cystitis.[18]

Rituximab (Rituxan)

- Rituximab is a monoclonal antibody that targets CD20 on the surface of B lymphocytes and reduces the number of B cells[7] (Figure 7.10).
- Several studies have shown a significant reduction in MS and neuromyelitis optica (NMO) relapses as well as in MRI activity.[3]
- This agent may increase the risk of infections, allergic reactions, cardiac arrhythmias, and cytopenias. Rare cases of PML have been reported.[6]

Mycophenolate Mofetil (CellCept)

- Mycophenolate mofetil, an inhibitor of inosine monophosphate dehydrogenase (IMPDH), inhibits de novo nucleotide synthesis and halts proliferation of T and B lymphocytes[19] (Figure 7.13).

METHOTREXATE

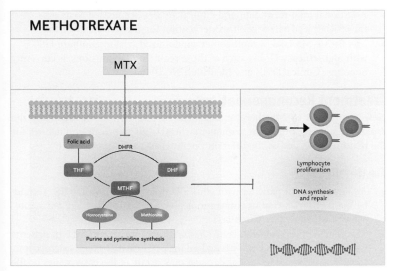

Figure 7.14 Mechanism of action of methotrexate. Abbreviations: DHF, dihydrofolate; MTHF, methyl tetrahydrofolate; MTX, methotrexate; THF, tetrahydrofolate.

- Results from clinical studies suggest that this agent may reduce relapse rates in MS and may slow disease worsening.[3]
- Side effects include increased risk of infection (including opportunistic infections such as PML), nausea, diarrhea, weakness, stomach ulcers, jaundice, and increased risk of skin cancer and lymphoma.[3]

Methotrexate

- Methotrexate is a folate antimetabolite that inhibits DNA synthesis, repair, and cellular replication, including that of T and B lymphocytes[18] (Figure 7.14).
- It has been shown to decrease the number of relapses in patients with MS and NMO, although its effectiveness compared to other standard DMTs is unclear.[3]
- Side effects include gastrointestinal bleeding, joint pain, mouth sores, and lower-extremity swelling.[18]

Stem Cell Transplantation

- The ultimate goal of autologous hematopoietic stem cell transplantation (HSCT) is to eliminate and replace the patient's pathogenic immune system, thereby achieving long-term remission of MS.[20]

- Additional long-term data and clinical studies are needed to assess the efficacy and safety of this intervention for the treatment of MS.[6]
- The BEAT-MS trial, a multicenter randomized trial to compare HSCT with high-efficacy DMTs such as those requiring IV infusions, is currently ongoing (ClinicalTrials.gov identifier: NCT04047628).

Treatment Recommendations

New approaches to MS therapy and goals of care have been driven by the rapidly expanding treatment armamentarium. Clinical practice guidelines for the treatment MS across its different phenotypes are discussed next.

Treatment of CIS

- Acute relapses in patients with clinically isolated syndrome (CIS) should be managed with oral or intravenous glucocorticoids, just like any acute MS exacerbation (see Chapter 1).
- The results of randomized controlled trials support early DMT in patients with CIS.[21–24] This is largely based on the premise that silent, microscopic, as well as irreversible axonal damage may occur in the early stages of the disease, and early treatment can help improve long-term outcomes by delaying time to accrued disability.[4]
- DMTs with evidence of efficacy for CIS include interferons, glatiramer acetate, teriflunomide, and (in the United States) siponimod.[21–26]
- Although the benefits of early CIS treatment for improving prognosis are not firmly established at this time, the authors of this book believe that early treatment of CIS (once a diagnosis is clear and other possible MS mimics have been ruled out) is likely to have a greater impact on delaying disease progression to MS and reducing long-term disability.

Treatment of RRMS

- All patients with a definite diagnosis of relapsing-remitting MS (RRMS) or with a first episode of neurologic symptoms and MRI findings consistent with MS should begin DMT.[3]
- It is important to keep in mind that DMTs are not a cure. Instead, their use is intended to reduce new lesions on MRI and consequently relapse rates, possibly reducing disease progression.
- DMTs should be continued indefinitely, but a switch to a different DMT should be considered in the following situations:[3]
    . The treatment fails to adequately control the disease based on clinical or MRI activity.
    . The side effects are intolerable to the patient.

- The patient is unable to comply with the treatment.
- A more appropriate treatment becomes available.

- Important exceptions to indefinite use of DMT include natalizumab therapy, where the risk of PML increases with the duration of treatment, and pregnancy, where the risk of adverse effects to the fetus must be weighed against discontinuation of therapy.[7]
- In general, the choice of a specific DMT agent should be individualized according to disease activity and patient preferences.[1]

    - The injectable agents (interferons or glatiramer acetate) can be used in patients who value safety more than effectiveness and convenience and in patients with mild to moderate disease.
    - Oral medications (dimethyl fumarate, teriflunomide, or fingolimod) can be used in patients who value convenience and have mild to moderate disease.
    - Infusion therapies and HSCT are usually reserved for patients with more aggressive disease (brainstem or spinal cord involvement and high lesion load on MRI) and for those who value effectiveness above safety and convenience.

Treatment of SPMS

- For patients with RRMS who reach the stage of secondary progressive MS (SPMS), particularly those with active disease defined either clinically or by MRI, treatment options include continuing the same DMT used during the RRMS phase or switching to a different DMT.[27,28]
- Siponimod (Mayzent) and cladribine (Mavenclad) have been FDA approved for the treatment of SPMS with relapses (active). Relapses are associated with more rapid progression of disability.[28]
- Discontinuation of DMT can be considered in patients with no ongoing relapses or MRI activity who have not been ambulatory for at least two years.[3]

Treatment of PPMS

- Ocrelizumab is the only FDA-approved DMT for use in patients with primary progressive MS (PPMS) at this time due to its ability to reduce the risk of disability progression in these patients.[10] Use of other DMTs for PPMS is empiric, as they lack convincing clinical trial evidence for effectiveness at this time.
- Clinical trials have not evaluated the benefits of DMT in nonambulatory patients with respect to other clinically relevant domains such as vision, cognition, and upper limb function.[3]

Treatment of RIS

- There are no official practice guidelines regarding the management of patients with radiologically isolated syndrome (RIS). Current evidence does not support initiation of DMT in these patients, even when the radiographic findings suggest subclinical MS.[29]

- The use of DMT in RIS is not routinely recommended outside of clinical trials.

DMT Use in Pregnancy

- Routine monitoring of the reproductive plans of all women with MS is essential.[7]

- Clinicians should provide appropriate counseling regarding reproductive risks and use of birth control during DMT use in all women with MS who are of reproductive age.

- Because DMTs may pose potential risks to the fetus to varying degrees, these treatments should not be started during pregnancy unless the risk of MS activity during pregnancy outweighs the risks associated with the specific DMT.[3]

- If accidental exposure to a DMT does occur during pregnancy, the DMT should be discontinued unless the risk of MS activity during pregnancy outweighs the risks associated with the specific DMT.[3]

- If a woman with MS is planning to become pregnant, clinicians should advise discontinuing DMT before conception unless the risk of MS activity during pregnancy outweighs the risks associated with the specific DMT.[3]

- None of the DMTs has received FDA approval for use during pregnancy or breastfeeding. Glatiramer acetate has not been associated with spontaneous abortions, complications during pregnancy, or birth defects, but like all other DMTs it should be avoided during lactation.

Future Therapies

A number of clinical trials have been listed in the National Institutes of Health (NIH) registry, which can be accessed at www.clinicaltrials.gov. In this section, we discuss a few promising drugs that were in Phase III clinical trials at the time of this book's writing.

BTK Modulation

- **Evobrutinib**
  - Clinicaltrials.gov identifiers: NCT04032158, NCT04032171.
  - Under investigation as treatment for RRMS.
  - This drug interferes with macrophage function, which has been linked to progression in MS as well as to increased activity of B cells. It works

by inhibiting Bruton's tyrosine kinase (BTK), an enzyme involved in the activation of B cells and macrophages.

. Evobrutinib is taken as a twice-daily oral tablet.

. In patients with RRMS, evobrutinib has shown a reduced number of new active lesions on MRI, in addition to reducing yearly relapse rates.

. In a Phase II study of 267 patients with RRMS, patients taking evobrutinib were compared to patients taking either placebo or dimethyl fumarate.[30]

  – The primary outcome measure was the number of active lesions on MRI.

  – When assessed 24 weeks after treatment, patients who initially took evobrutinib were found to have significantly fewer active lesions compared to those in the placebo group.

. A common side effect reported in Phase II clinical trials was transaminitis.

. EVOLUTION RMS1 and RMS2 are two identical Phase III clinical studies that will recruit 1,900 patients with RRMS. Half of the patients will be randomized to either an evobrutinib or an Avonex (interferon beta-1a) group and will be receive the same treatment for approximately 2 years.

Anti-CD20 Monoclonal Antibodies

• **Ofatumumab**

  . Clinicaltrials.gov identifier: NCT03650114.

  . Under investigation as treatment for RRMS.

  . This drug reduces the number of B lymphocytes.

  . It is a monoclonal antibody that binds CD20 (a B cell surface marker) and causes targeted destruction of B cells.

  . Ofatumumab is currently used to treat chronic lymphocytic leukemia (CML).

  . It is taken as a subcutaneous injection every 4 weeks.

  . Thus far, the results of Phase II trials comparing the efficacy of ofatumumab against placebo have shown a 65% reduction in new active MRI lesions within a 24-week treatment period.[31]

  . Preliminary results from Phase III studies (ASCLEPIOS I and ASCLEPIOS II) in which ofatumumab was compared to teriflunomide show that ofatumumab reduced relapses by 50% to 59% and reduced the risk of disability progression by about 30% compared to teriflunomide.[32,33]

  . The most frequent side effect reported was injection-site reactions.

- **Ublituximab**

  - Clinicaltrials.gov identifier: NCT03277261.
  - Under investigation as treatment for RRMS.
  - This drug reduces the number of B lymphocytes.
  - It is a monoclonal antibody that binds CD20 (a B cell surface marker) and causes targeted destruction of B cells.
  - In clinical trials, ublituximab was given as an intravenous infusion on day 1, day 15, and week 24.
  - Results of Phase II studies in 48 patients with RRMS showed that ublituximab reduced overall MRI lesion volume by 10% at week 48, and 93% of patients were relapse-free during the entirety of the study.[34]
  - Ongoing Phase III studies (ULTIMATE 1 and ULTIMATE 2) will compare the efficacy of ublituximab to that of teriflunomide. The primary outcome of the study will be the number of relapses each participant has every year.
  - The most frequent side effect reported was infusion-related reactions.

Sphingosine-1-Phosphate Receptor Modulators

- **Ozanimod**

  - Clinicaltrials.gov identifier: NCT02576717.
  - Awaiting approval by the FDA and the European Medicines Agency (EMA) as treatment for RRMS.
  - This drug binds to the sphingosine-1-phosphate receptor and results in retention of lymphocytes within lymph nodes, preventing their migration into the central nervous system.
  - It is taken as an oral tablet once per day.
  - In a Phase III study (SUNBEAM), ozanimod reduced relapse rates by about 48% compared to beta interferon.[35]
  - In another Phase III study (RADIANCE), ozanimod reduced relapse rates by about 38% compared to beta interferon.[36]
  - In both Phase III studies, ozanimod significantly reduced the number of new active lesions on MRI.
  - The most common side effects reported are flu-like symptoms and urinary tract infections.

- **Ponesimod**

  - Clinicaltrials.gov identifier: NCT02907177.
  - Under investigation as treatment for RRMS.
  - This drug binds to the sphingosine-1-phosphate receptor and results in retention of lymphocytes within lymph nodes, preventing their migration into the central nervous system.

- It is taken as an oral tablet once per day.
- In a Phase III clinical study (OPTIMUM), ponesimod reduced relapse rates by about 30% and reduced the number of active lesions on brain MRI by 56% compared to teriflunomide.[36]
- In another Phase III study (POINT), participants will take either ponesimod or placebo in addition to dimethyl fumarate for at least 60 weeks.

  - The primary outcome of the study will be relapse-rate reduction. The study will also measure disability progression, effects on brain volume, time to first relapse, disease activity on MRI scans, fatigue, and adverse events.

- The most common side effects reported are anxiety, dizziness, transaminitis, insomnia, and peripheral edema (lower extremity swelling).

Tyrosine Kinase Inhibition
- **Masitinib**
  - Clinicaltrials.gov identifier: NCT01433497.
  - Under investigation as treatment for RRMS, SPMS, and PPMS.
  - This drug inhibits tyrosine kinase, an enzyme involved in inflammation and immune responses. It targets mast cells.
  - It is an oral tablet taken twice daily.
  - In a Phase II study, 35 patients with primary and secondary MS were randomized to placebo or masitinib for 18 months.[37]

    - Patients in the masitinib arm showed an improvement in the MS functional composite (MFSC) score, which assesses walking ability, hand and arm coordination, and mental function.
    - Patients in the placebo group showed worsening in the MSFC score.
    - The results were not statistically significant.

  - Further research is planned in a larger study in the United States and France, which will randomize 450 patients into masitinib or placebo for 20 months.

    - The primary endpoint of the study will be MSFC score.

  - The most common side effects reported were asthenia, rash, nausea, edema, and diarrhea.

Biotin
- **MD1003**
  - Clinicaltrials.gov identifier: NCT02936037.

- Under investigation as treatment for SPMS and PPMS.
- Biotin activates key enzymes involved in cell growth, energy production, and myelin synthesis and is thought to have an impact on disability and progression in MS.
- This is a highly concentrated formulation of biotin taken as a 100-mg capsule three times per day.
- MS-ON was a Phase III trial that compared MD1003 to placebo in treating chronic visual loss related to optic neuritis in MS.[37]

  - Patients taking MD1003 improved slightly more compared to those in the placebo group, but there was no statistical significance.

- SPI2 is a study that will compare MD1003 or placebo in approximately 300 patients with SPMS or PPMS.

  - The primary endpoint will be improvement in disability, defined as either a lower EDSS score or a reduction in the time to walk 25 feet.

- The most common side effects reported were urinary tract infections and headache.

Statin Therapy

- **Simvastatin**

  - Clinicaltrials.gov identifier: NCT00647348.
  - Under investigation as treatment for SPMS.
  - The exact mechanism of simvastatin in MS is not known, but it has shown to reduce brain atrophy and slow down progression of the disease. It is also thought to have some neuroprotective effects.
  - The MS-STAT1 clinical trial randomized patients with SPMS into placebo or simvastatin for 2 years.[37]

    - In the treatment group, brain atrophy was reduced by 43% compared to placebo.
    - There was also a slower change in EDSS and improved MSIS-29 questionnaire, which measures the effect of MS on daily life.

  - MS-STAT2 is a Phase III study that will further investigate the potential effects of simvastatin on SPMS.
  - Common reported side effects include nosebleeds, sore throat, headache, nausea, gastrointestinal problems, and muscle and joint pain.

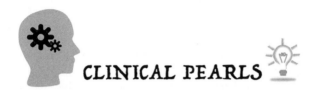

CLINICAL PEARLS

- Early and ongoing treatment with a disease-modifying agent in MS is essential to reduce ongoing disease and delay progression of disability.
- Having realistic expectations and considering patient preference regarding the different modalities of treatment (injectables, oral agents, or infusion therapies) can help ensure treatment adherence and compliance.
- Medication side effects and costs should also be kept in mind when choosing a disease-modifying agent.
- Sequential MRI surveillance is important after starting a DMT to ensure treatment efficacy and determine the need for escalation therapy.
- BTK, tyrosine kinase, and sphingosine-1-phosphate receptor modulators, as well as highly concentrated biotin and statins, are currently under investigation for treatment of relapsing and progressive forms of MS.

References

1. Cross AH, Naismith RT. Established and novel disease-modifying treatments in multiple sclerosis. *J Intern Med.* 2014;275(4):350–63. doi:10.1111/joim.12203

2. Tillery EE, Clements JN, Howard Z. What's new in multiple sclerosis? *Ment Heal Clin.* 2017;7(5):213–20. doi:10.9740/mhc.2017.09.213

3. Rae-Grant A, Day GS, Marrie RA, et al. Practice guideline recommendations summary: disease-modifying therapies for adults with multiple sclerosis. *Neurology.* 2018;90(17):777–88. doi:10.1212/WNL.0000000000005347

4. Kappos L, Freedman MS, Polman CH, et al. Long-term effect of early treatment with interferon beta-1b after a first clinical event suggestive of multiple sclerosis: 5-year active treatment extension of the phase 3 BENEFIT trial. *Lancet Neurol.* 2009;8(11):987–97. doi:10.1016/S1474-4422(09)70237-6

5. Marcus JF, Waubant EL. Updates on clinically isolated syndrome and diagnostic criteria for multiple sclerosis. *Neurohospitalist.* 2013;3(2):65–80. doi:10.1177/1941874412457183

6. Eriksson I, Komen J, Piehl F, et al. The changing multiple sclerosis treatment landscape: impact of new drugs and treatment recommendations. *Eur J Clin Pharmacol.* 2018;74:663–70. doi:10.1007/s00228-018-2429-1

7. Wingerchuk DM, Carter JL. Multiple sclerosis: current and emerging disease-modifying therapies and treatment strategies. *Mayo Clin Proc.* 2014;89(2):225–40. doi:10.1016/j.mayocp.2013.11.002

8. Olek MJ. Differential diagnosis, clinical features, and prognosis of multiple sclerosis. *Curr Clin Neurol Mult Scler.* 2005:15–53.

9. Jones DE. Early relapsing multiple sclerosis. *Continuum (Minneap Minn).* 2016;22(3):744–60. doi:10.1212/CON.0000000000000329

10. Ciotti JR, Cross AH. Disease-modifying treatment in progressive multiple sclerosis. *Curr Treat Options Neurol.* 2018;20(5):12. doi:10.1007/s11940-018-0496-3

11. Dumitrescu L, Constantinescu CS, Tanasescu R. Siponimod for the treatment of secondary progressive multiple sclerosis. *Expert Opin Pharmacother.* 2018;20 (2):143–50.

12. Food and Drug Administration. FDA approves new oral treatment for multiple sclerosis.

13. Neema M, Stankiewicz J, Arora A, et al. MRI in multiple sclerosis: what's inside the toolbox? *Neurotherapeutics.* 2007;4:602–17. doi:10.1016/j.nurt.2007.08.001

14. Rocca MA, Messina R, Filippi M. Multiple sclerosis imaging: recent advances. *J Neurol.* 2013;260(3):929–35. doi:10.1007/s00415-012-6788-8

15. Feinstein A, Freeman J, Lo AC. Treatment of progressive multiple sclerosis: what works, what does not, and what is needed. *Lancet Neurol.* 2015;14(2):194–207.

16. Ching B, Mohamed A, Khoo T, Ismail H. Multiphasic disseminated encephalomyelitis followed by optic neuritis in a child with gluten sensitivity. *Mult Scler J.* 2015;21(9):1209–11. doi:10.1177/

17. Wingerchuk DM. Immune-mediated myelopathies. *Continuum (Minneap Minn).* 2018;24(2):497–522. doi:10.1212/CON.0000000000000582

18. Freedman MS, Rush CA. Severe, highly active, or aggressive multiple sclerosis. *Continuum (Minneap Minn).* 2016;22(3):761–84. doi:10.1212/CON.0000000000000331

19. Hacohen Y, Wong YY, Lechner C, et al. Disease course and treatment responses in children with relapsing myelin oligodendrocyte glycoprotein antibody–associated disease. *JAMA Neurol.* 2018;75(4):478–87. doi:10.1001/jamaneurol.2017.4601

20. Thompson AJ, Baranzini SE, Geurts J, et al. Multiple sclerosis. *Lancet Neurol.* 2018;391:1622–36. doi:10.1016/B978-0-7234-3748-2.00015-3

21. Hauser SL, Bar-Or A, Cohen J, et al. Ofatumumab versus teriflunomide in relapsing MS: adaptive design of two Phase 3 studies (ASCLEPIOS I and ASCLEPIOS II) (S16.005). *Neurology.* 2017;88(16 suppl):S16.005. http://n.neurology.org/content/88/16_Supplement/S16.005.abstract.

22. Fox E, Wray S, Shubin R, et al. Open label extension (OLE) of Phase 2 multicenter study of ublituximab (UTX), a novel glycoengineered anti-CD20 monoclonal antibody (mAb), in patients with relapsing forms of multiple sclerosis (RMS) (P3.2-048). *Neurology*. 2019;92(15 suppl):P3.2-048. http://n.neurology.org/content/92/15_Supplement/P3.2-048.abstract.

23. Comi G, Kappos L, Selmaj KW, et al. Safety and efficacy of ozanimod versus interferon beta-1a in relapsing multiple sclerosis (SUNBEAM): a multicentre, randomised, minimum 12-month, phase 3 trial. *Lancet Neurol*. 2019;18 (11):1009–20. doi:10.1016/S1474-4422(19)30239-X

24. Cohen JA, Comi G, Selmaj KW, et al. Safety and efficacy of ozanimod versus interferon beta-1a in relapsing multiple sclerosis (RADIANCE): a multicentre, randomised, 24-month, phase 3 trial. *Lancet Neurol*. 2019;18(11):1021–33. doi:10.1016/S1474-4422(19)30238-8

25. Vermersch P, Benrabah R, Schmidt N, et al. Masitinib treatment in patients with progressive multiple sclerosis: a randomized pilot study. *BMC Neurol*. 2012;12:36. doi:10.1186/1471-2377-12-36

26. Willis M, Fox R. Progressive multiple sclerosis. *Continuum (Minneap Minn)*. 2016;22(3):785–98.

27. Eriksson M, Andersen O, Runmarker B. Long-term follow up of patients with clinically isolated syndromes, relapsing-remitting and secondary progressive multiple sclerosis. *Mult Scler*. 2003;9:260–74.

28. Cree BAC, Gourraud PA, Oksenberg JR, et al. Long-term evolution of multiple sclerosis disability in the treatment era. *Ann Neurol*. 2016;80(4):499–510. doi:10.1002/ana.24747

29. Granberg T, Martola J, Kristoffersen-Wiberg M, et al. Radiologically isolated syndrome: incidental magnetic resonance imaging findings suggestive of multiple sclerosis, a systematic review. *Mult Scler J*. 2013;19(3):271–80. doi:10.1177/1352458512451943

30. Montalban X, Arnold DL, Weber MS, et al. Placebo-controlled trial of an oral BTK inhibitor in multiple sclerosis. *N Engl J Med*. 2019;380(25):2406–17. doi:10.1056/NEJMoa1901981

31. Sorensen PS, Lisby S, Grove R, et al. Safety and efficacy of ofatumumab in relapsing-remitting multiple sclerosis. *Neurology*. 2014;82(7):573–81. doi:10.1212/WNL.0000000000000125

32. Kish T. Promising multiple sclerosis agents in late-stage development. *PT*. 2018;43 (12):750–72. www.ncbi.nlm.nih.gov/pubmed/30559588.

Chapter 8

Treatment Goals

Andrew Smith, MD

Introduction

The goals of treatment in multiple sclerosis (MS) have evolved greatly over the past few decades. The original natural history of MS cohorts described in Olmsted County, Minnesota, and in Lyon, France, suggested that MS patients became disabled around the same age regardless of treatment.[1,2] Therefore, even after the development of disease-modifying therapies (DMTs), the concept of medical futility remained in the field.

Over time, data has accumulated supporting the notion of a "treatment window" in which the course of disease can be altered.

- Long-term data from the pivotal DMT studies suggested a long-term benefit of treatment.[3]
- More recently, multiple clinical trials involving patients with clinically isolated syndrome (CIS) have shown the benefit of early treatment in slowing the transition to clinically definite MS (CDMS).[3-6]

Consequently, the field has shifted in favor of early treatment in MS care.

The Case for Early Treatment

- The primary goal of treatment in MS is to delay disease progression and limit disability over time by reducing the inflammatory component of the disease.[7]
- Evidence from large epidemiological studies and clinical trials suggests that this window of opportunity closes relatively early in the disease course, defined as an Expanded Disability Status Scale (EDSS) score of 3 or less[8-10] (see Appendix 1).

  - Prior to reaching an EDSS score of 3.0, incomplete recovery from relapses drives disability accumulation.

- After reaching an EDSS score of 3.0, neurodegeneration occurs and neurologic deterioration may progress at a set rate, though this varies among patients.[8]
- Regardless of the disease phenotype, the time for a patient with an EDSS score of 3.0 to reach 6.5 (walking with bilateral assistance) is fairly consistent (12 years).[9]

Treatment Approaches

While early treatment has become the norm in MS, there is current debate as to which therapeutic agent should be initiated first. While this is a large oversimplification, three types of strategies are used to treat MS: escalation, induction, and early use of highly effective medication. While arguments can be made for each of these approaches, treatment should always be tailored to each patient on an individual basis. In the real world, different providers may use different strategies, or a combination of them. The approach that each provider ultimately choses for a patient should generally depend on the severity of the patient's disease. Most importantly, anecdotally, lack of appropriate long-term monitoring (clinical and radiological) plays an important role in accumulation of irreversible disability.

Escalation

- The escalation approach favors the initiation of the injectable therapies, which are considered "platform" or first-line drugs (Figure 8.1).
  - These are oldest and most well-studied therapies.
  - They are also considered the safest DMTs.
  - According to this approach, platform therapies should be escalated to a higher-efficacy agent only if treatment with the first-line agent fails.
  - A common argument for this approach is largely based on concerns over unnecessary exposure of patients to the complex safety profiles of the high-efficacy DMTs.
  - Critics of this approach suggest that failing to control the disease at its earlier stages will inevitably result in worse long-term outcomes.

Induction

- The induction approach favors the use of more aggressive, higher-efficacy DMTs as first-line therapy over a short period of time (a few months to 2 years), after which it is replaced by an agent with moderate efficacy (Figure 8.2).
- The rationale behind the induction approach that initial aggressive can help delay progression to the more chronic phases of the disease, which ultimately lead to irreversible disability. In other words, if the least

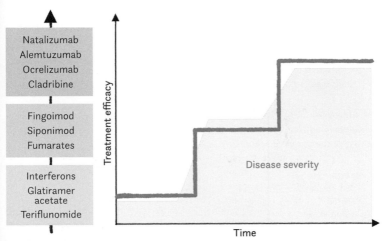

Figure 8.1 Escalation approach to treatment of MS. This approach favors the initiation of platform (less efficacious) therapy with escalation to higher-efficacy agents only if treatment with first-line agents fails.

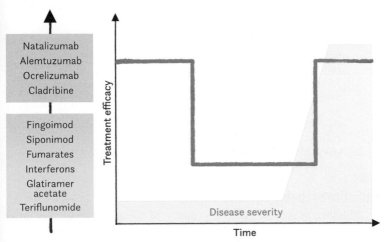

Figure 8.2 Induction approach to treatment of MS. This approach favors the initiation of high-efficacy agents at onset over a period of months to a few years, after which they are replaced by a moderate-efficacy agent.

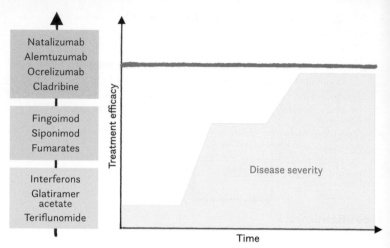

Figure 8.3 Early use of highly efficacious therapy approach to treatment of MS. This approach favors the use of high-efficacy drugs as first-line treatment from disease onset.

effective treatments are used initially, the therapeutic window may be missed, putting the patient at risk of treatment failure with the possibility of early disability accumulation.[10]

- The possible risk of missing the treatment window is considered even higher in those individuals who have a more aggressive disease course early on.[11]
- Providers who adhere to this approach argue that MS is not as benign as many would think, with most patients developing significant disability and employability issues within 20 years after their diagnosis.
- Critics argue that exposing patients to high-risk medications that may not improve the long-term course of the disease may not outweigh the benefits of therapy.

Early Use of Highly Effective Therapy

- This therapy approach generally consists of the use of high-efficacy drugs as first-line treatment, and continuing treatment with these agents in the long run without switching to less effective therapies (Figure 8.3).
- Similar to the induction approach, this approach argues against the use of platform therapies as first-line due to the concerns of inefficacy.

- Critics argue that more aggressive therapies should be used as first-line treatment only in patients with evidence of aggressive disease, either clinically or on follow-up magnetic resonance imaging (MRI) scans, or both.

    - Risk factors for aggressive disease include male gender, non-white race, initial attacks with motor deficits or ataxia, incomplete relapse recovery, early second relapse, brainstem and spinal cord involvement on MRI, and high total T2 and enhancing T1 lesion burden on initial MRI.

- Practitioners who follow the escalation approach would argue that starting with high-efficacy medication may put the patient at higher risk of unnecessary side effects.
- Those in favor of the induction approach would argue that this group could also potentially miss the therapeutic window.

Treatment Goals

- Regardless of the specific therapy approach followed, *the primary goal of MS treatment is to decrease clinical and radiologic disease activity so as to avoid accumulation of irreversible disability over time, while minimizing the negative impact of the potential side effects.*
- Currently, practitioners rely on clinical and radiographic assessments to determine ongoing disease activity and response to treatment.
- Determining the response to treatment is a trial-and-error process. Because response to DMTs varies among patients, identifying those with suboptimal therapy responses as early as possible is essential. Therefore, close clinical monitoring is important in all patients with recent therapy initiation or therapy switch.
- Newly diagnosed patients should be seen for follow-up at months 3, 6, and 12 after initiating therapy, and MRI should be repeated at month 6 or 12 depending on the DMT selected. Preferably, scans should be obtained by using the same scanner and/or same field strength as for the initial MRI.

Determining Treatment Response

- Two main treatment strategies are helpful in assessing patient response to therapy: the modified Rio score and the concept of no evidence of disease activity (NEDA).

    - They differ in terms of how much disease activity is allowed before one declares a disease modifying therapy a failure.
    - The most commonly used measure is the modified Rio score (see Appendix 4), which allows for some disease activity prior to considering failure of a specific treatment.

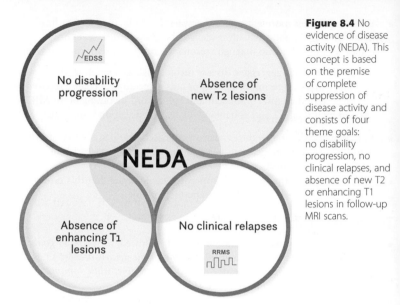

Figure 8.4 No evidence of disease activity (NEDA). This concept is based on the premise of complete suppression of disease activity and consists of four theme goals: no disability progression, no clinical relapses, and absence of new T2 or enhancing T1 lesions in follow-up MRI scans.

- The concept of NEDA is focused on complete suppression of disease activity.

    - In progressive MS, this is referred to as no evidence of progression or active disease (NEPAD).

- The overarching theme of these goals is to ensure there is no detectable evidence of MS disease activity.

No Evidence of Disease Activity

The concept of NEDA emerged from the AFFRIM trial, a Phase III clinical trial of natalizumab. A post-hoc analysis of this trial by Havrdova et al.[12] demonstrated that 37% of natalizumab-treated patients had no evidence of either radiographic or clinical disease activity at follow-up (Figure 8.4). This condition was initially referred to as "disease activity free" (DAF), but the term has evolved into what is now known as NEDA-3.

- NEDA-3

    1. Consists of three main goals:[13]

        - Absence of clinical relapses
        - No sustained disability progression as measured by EDSS score

Table 8.1 No evidence of disease activity (NEDA)[12,15]

NEDA-3	1. No clinical relapses 2. No sustained disability progression 3. No gadolinium-enhancing lesions and no new or enlarging T2-hyperintense lesions on cranial MRI
NEDA-4	1. No clinical relapses 2. No sustained disability progression 3. No gadolinium-enhancing lesions and no new or enlarging T2-hyperintense lesions on cranial MRI 4. Brain volume atrophy less than 0.4%

- No MRI activity, described as presence of new or enlarged T2 lesions compared to a previous scan or new active (enhanced) lesions on post-gadolinium T1 scan

2. NEDA-3 is commonly used by specialists in the clinic setting.

- NEDA-4

1. Some argue NEDA-3 does not accurately predict MS outcomes.
2. The NEDA-3 concept lacks a sensitive measure of disability progression and neurodegeneration.

- About half of the patients achieving NEDA may develop cognitive decline at two years.[14]

3. To improve the definition of NEDA-3, brain volume loss of less than 0.4% per year was added as a marker of neurodegeneration.
4. This became known as NEDA-4.

- NEDA-4 is generally used only in research settings due to the inability of most centers to measure brain atrophy in the clinic setting.

- Beyond NEDA-4

1. As with NEDA-3, some argue that the NEDA-4 concept does not accurately predict MS outcomes (Table 8.1 summarizes NEDA-3 and NEDA-4 criteria).

- They argue that other measures, such as cognitive outcomes and serum neurofilament light chain (NfL) measurements, should be added to NEDA to increase its sensitivity.

- The major criticisms of NEDA are twofold:

    1. The difficulty of successfully achieving NEDA.

        – In an ideal setting, NEDA is achieved less than half of the time (mostly due to the intrinsic therapeutic limitations of DMTs).
        – Only 10% of patients who achieve NEDA are able to maintain this state 8 years later.[16,17]

    2. Whether achieving NEDA matters.

        – Achieving NEDA for the first two years has not clearly demonstrated an improvement in clinical outcomes 7–10 years later.[18–22]
        – Critics argue that chasing the goal of NEDA:
            ○ Can lead to endless escalation of therapy
            ○ Can result in increased exposure to potential side effects
            ○ Is unachievable on a long-term basis
            ○ Does not guarantee better clinical outcomes
        – Despite these criticisms, NEDA-3 is the current gold standard treatment goal in RRMS.

No Evidence of Progression or Active Disease

The concept of NEPAD is relatively new and developed as a treatment goal for progressive forms of MS from the INFORMS and ORATORIO trials.[13,22] The concept of NEPAD marries the concept of no active disease, as measured by clinical relapses or MRI lesions, with methods of detecting disability progression. NEPAD introduced a new treatment goal of no evidence of progression (NEP). Table 8.2 summarizes the definitions of NEP and NEPAD.

- NEP: [13,22]

    . The criticism of NEPAD is similar to that faced by NEDA-3.

Indications for Switching DMTs

- While the Rio score and NEDA are convenient ways to measure disability progression, there is no correct answer to the question of when to declare treatment failure.
- The extremes are simpler. Most MS specialists:

    . Would not switch a DMT in a patient with **one** new T2 lesion or **one** relapse over a decade in a patient who has tolerated the medication well.
    . Would likely switch DMTs in a patient with **more than two** new T2 lesions (or one enhancing T1 lesion) on MRI or if the patient relapsed once **within 5 years of diagnosis**.

Table 8.2 No evidence of progression (NEP) and no evidence of progression and no evidence of progression and active disease (NEDAP) definitions[13,14]

NEP	1. No 12-week confirmed disability progression, defined as:
	a. An increase of 1 point in those with an EDSS score less than or equal to 5.5
	b. An increase of 0.5 point in those with an EDSS score greater than 5.5
	2. No 12-week confirmed 20% increase in time for the 25-foot walk test time
	3. No 12-week confirmed 20% increase on the 9-hole peg test (9-HPT) score
NEDAP	1. No relapses on treatment
	2. No 12-week disability progression on EDSS score
	3. No confirmed disability progression of 20% or more in 9-HPT score
	4. No confirmed disability progression of 20% or more in 25-foot walk test time
	5. No new or enlarging T2 MRI lesions and no gadolinium-enhancing T1 lesions

- Would debate changing the medication if a patient:
  - Has a new T2 lesion at the first follow-up MRI after starting a DMT.
  - Develops one or two new lesions in one MRI but repeat MRIs after 6 months are stable.
  - Has a relapse that could not be documented by neurologic exam and is patient-reported only.

- However, it is important to take into account the full clinical context of each individual patient when making a decision on whether a DMT should be switched.
- Most importantly, MRI comparison should be done by the physician making the decision to switch DMT. Scans are best compared when obtained in the same scanner at the same magnet strength. Comparing different protocols and magnet strengths (e.g., 1.5T versus 3T) may cause detection of lesions that may appear as new based on technique, head position, or increased magnet strength.

Conclusion

Controversy exists about what the ultimate treatment goals in MS should be. Nevertheless, available evidence suggests that the disease should be treated as early as possible, as long as the diagnosis is clearly stablished. It is important to consider many potential factors before starting or changing DMTs. In addition to effectiveness, clinicians should consider patient preferences and goals of therapy. Failure to take patient considerations into account when making treatment decisions can compromise medication compliance and lead to decreased patient satisfaction rates.[22]

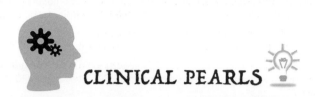

CLINICAL PEARLS

- The primary goal of treatment in MS is to delay disease progression and limit disability over time by reducing the inflammatory component of the disease.
- Treatment strategies in MS fall into three categories: escalation, induction, and early use of highly effective therapy.
- Medication side effects and costs should also be kept in mind when choosing a disease-modifying agent.
- Regardless of the specific therapy approach followed, the primary goal of treatment is to decrease clinical and radiologic disease activity so as to avoid accumulation of irreversible disability over time.

References

1. Mayr WT, Pittock SJ, McClelland RL, et al. Incidence and prevalence of multiple sclerosis in Olmsted County, Minnesota, 1985–2000. *Neurology.* 2003;61(10):1373–7.

2. Confavreux C, Vukusic S, Moreau T, Adeleine P. Relapses and progression of disability in multiple sclerosis. *N Engl J Med.* 2000;343(20):1430–8.

3. Bruck W, Stadelmann C. Inflammation and degeneration in multiple sclerosis. J Neurol Sci. 2003;24(suppl 5):S265–7.

4. McKay KA, Kwan V, Duggan T, Tremlett H. Risk factors associated with the onset of relapsing-remitting and primary progressive multiple sclerosis: a systematic review. Biomed Res Int. 2015;2015:817238.

5. Leray E, Yaouanq J, Le Page E, et al. Evidence for a two-stage disability progression in multiple sclerosis. *Brain.* 2010;133(Pt 7):1900–13.

6. Confavreux C, Vukusic S, Adeleine P. Early clinical predictors and progression of irreversible disability in multiple sclerosis: an amnesic process. *Brain.* 2003;126(Pt 4):770–82.

7. Kappos L, Edan G, Freedman MS, et al. The 11-year long-term follow-up study from the randomized BENEFIT CIS trial. *Neurology.* 2016;87(10):978–87.

8. Hua LH, Fan TH, Conway D, et al. Discontinuation of disease-modifying therapy in patients with multiple sclerosis over age 60. *Mult Scler.* 2018:1352458518765656.

9. MS F. Multiple sclerosis therapeutic strategies: use second-line agents as first-line agents when time is of the essence. *Neurol Clin Pract.* 2011;1(1):66–8.

10. Damasceno A, Damasceno BP, Cendes F. No evidence of disease activity in multiple sclerosis: implications on cognition and brain atrophy. *Mult Scler.* 2016;22(1):64–72.

11. Uher T, Havrdova E, Sobisek L, et al. Is no evidence of disease activity an achievable goal in MS patients on intramuscular interferon beta-1a treatment over long-term follow-up? *Mult Scler.* 2017;23(2):242–52. doi:10.1177/1352458516650525

12. De Stefano N, Airas L, Grigoriadis N, et al. Clinical relevance of brain volume measures in multiple sclerosis. *CNS Drugs.* 2014;28(2):147–56.

13. Wolinsky JS, Montalban X, Hauser SL, et al. Evaluation of no evidence of progression or active disease (NEPAD) in patients with primary progressive multiple sclerosis in the ORATORIO trial. *Ann Neurol.* 2018;84(4):527–36.

14. Lublin F, Miller DH, Freedman MS, et al. Oral fingolimod in primary progressive multiple sclerosis (INFORMS): a Phase 3, randomised, double-blind, placebo-controlled trial. *Lancet.* 2016;387(10023):1075–84.

15. Havrdova E, Galetta S, Hutchinson M, et al. Effect of natalizumab on clinical and radiological disease activity in multiple sclerosis: a retrospective analysis of the Natalizumab Safety and Efficacy in Relapsing-Remitting Multiple Sclerosis (AFFIRM) study. *Lancet Neurol.* 2009;8(3):254-60.

16. Wattjes MP, Steenwijk MD, Stangel M. MRI in the diagnosis and monitoring of multiple sclerosis: an update. *Clin Neuroradiol.* 2015;25(suppl 2):157–65. doi:10.1007/s00062-015-0430-y

17. Pardo G, Jones DE. The sequence of disease-modifying therapies in relapsing multiple sclerosis: safety and immunologic considerations. *J Neurol.* 2017;264(12):2351–74. [Published correction appears in *J Neurol.* 2017;264(12):2375–77]. doi:10.1007/s00415-017-8594-9

18. Beck RW, Chandler DL, Cole SR, et al. Interferon beta-1a for early multiple sclerosis: CHAMPS trial subgroup analyses. *Ann Neurol.* 2002;51(4):481–90.

19. Comi G, Filippi M, Barkhof F, et al. Effect of early interferon treatment on conversion to definite multiple sclerosis: a randomised study. *Lancet.* 2001;357(9268):1576–82.

20. Kappos L, Edan G, Freedman MS, et al. The 11-year long-term follow-up study from the randomized BENEFIT CIS trial. *Neurology.* 2016;87(10):978–87.

21. Comi G, Martinelli V, Rodegher M, et al. Effect of glatiramer acetate on conversion to clinically definite multiple sclerosis in patients with clinically isolated syndrome (PreCISe study): a randomised double-blind, placebo-controlled trial. *Lancet.* 2009;374(9700)1503–11.

22. Degenhardt A, Ramagopalan SV, Scalfari A, et al. Clinical prognostic factors in multiple sclerosis: a natural history review. *Nat Rev Neurol.* 2009; 5: 672–82.

Symptomatic Management

Carlos A. Pérez, MD

Introduction

Symptoms of multiple sclerosis (MS) vary considerably from person to person and change over time. Most of these symptoms can be alleviated, but very few can be eliminated completely. Not all symptoms associated with MS are directly related to inflammation of the central nervous system. Although treatment of the disease itself is of major importance, treatment of secondary symptoms is equally important, as failure to do so can compromise quality of life for both patients and their families. In this chapter, we discuss the most common MS-related symptoms and their management. It is important to keep in mind that all treatments used have the potential for side effects. For some symptoms, nondrug approaches are the best initial approach to treatment. Potential difficulties associated with some forms of treatment are also discussed.

Bladder Dysfunction[1-4]

- **Common symptoms**

  . Urinary frequency, urgency, and nocturia.

- **Complications**

  . Urinary tract infections (UTI), particularly in women, may occur.

- **Types of bladder dysfunction** (Figure 9.1)

  . **Detrusor overactivity**

    – May result in urinary urgency, frequency, and urge incontinence.

  . **Neurogenic bladder or sphincter–detrusor dyssynergia**

    – May result in urinary retention, interrupted urination, and urinary frequency.

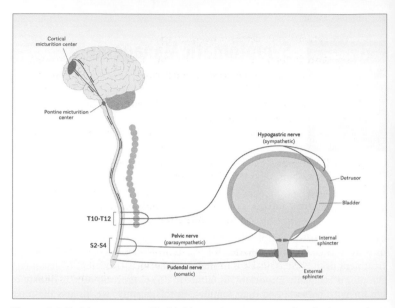

Figure 9.1 Bladder innervation. The bladder receives motor input from both sympathetic (hypogastric nerve) and parasympathetic (pelvic nerve) sources. Sensation from the bladder is transmitted to the micturition center in the brain, which then allows for voluntary control of the external sphincter via the pudendal nerve. Dyssynergia between any of these connections can lead to urinary incontinence. The hypogastric nerve acts on the internal sphincter via alpha-1 receptors. The pudendal nerve acts on the external sphincter via nicotinic acetylcholine receptors. (A black and white version of this figure will appear in some formats. For the colour version, please refer to the plate section.)

- **Clinical evaluation**

  - In males, prostate hypertrophy and urethral strictures may contribute to the symptoms.
  - Urinalysis may be performed to rule out an infectious cause.
  - In more severe cases, evaluation by a urologist should be performed. It may include:

    – Measurements of **post-void residual (PVR)** urine volume, which may indicate risk for renal calculi and hydronephrosis when elevated (typically more than 100 mL).
    – Urodynamic studies

- **Management**
  - For patients with **detrusor overactivity**:
    - **Anticholinergic and antimuscarinic drugs** are typically used.
      - ○ **Oxybutynin** decreases bladder emptying and consequently increases PVR.
      - ○ Other anticholinergic drugs include tolterodine, propantheline, and proviverrine.
      - ○ Common side effects include confusion, dry mouth, blurry vision, dizziness, and drowsiness.
    - **Botulinum toxin** (Botox) injections may be used in patients who are nonresponsive to drug therapy.
      - ○ Common side effects include urinary retention and urinary tract infections. In some cases, this may result in the need to initiate intermittent catheterization.
    - **Sacral neurostimulation**
      - ○ This modality is uncommonly used but may be useful in some patients unresponsive to drug therapy and/or botulinum toxin. This treatment inhibits the micturition reflex.
  - For patients with **failure to empty** (hypotonic neurogenic bladder or sphincter–detrusor dyssynergia)
    - **Alpha-antagonist medications** such as prazosin, terazosin, doxazosin, and tamsulosin may be used.
    - **Intermittent catheterization** may also be beneficial.
  - **Nondrug treatment**
    - Conservative management includes:
      - ○ Fluid restriction (generally to less than 2 L per day)
      - ○ Scheduled and regimented voiding
      - ○ Regular use of protective padding

Bowel Dysfunction[5,6]

- **Common symptoms**
  - Bowel dysfunction may result from upper and lower motor neuron impairment and may be divided into disorders of storage and elimination.

- **Complications**

  . Common symptoms may include constipation and incontinence.

- **Clinical evaluation**

  . Monitoring should be performed at each follow-up visit for all patients with MS.

- **Management**

  . **Constipation**

    – Dietary changes to include increased fluid intake and addition of dietary fiber.
    – Laxatives and enemas may also be used when dietary changes fail to improve the symptoms.
      ○ Examples of laxatives that may be used include magnesium sulfate, bisacodyl, senna, and docusate, among others.

  . **Fecal incontinence**

    – Initial management includes supportive care, including avoidance of foods or activities known to provoke symptoms.
    – Special attention should be paid to perianal skin hygiene to prevent other complications.
    – For patients who do not respond to conservative measures, additional evaluation via anorectal manometry and magnetic resonance imaging (MRI) should be performed by a gastroenterologist.
    – Some disease-modifying agents, such as dimethyl fumarate, may be associated with diarrhea and other gastrointestinal symptoms, and should be used with caution in patients with bowel incontinence.

Cognitive Impairment[7–10]

- **Common symptoms**

  . The cognitive domains most commonly affected in MS include:

    – Attention
    – Executive functioning
    – Short-term memory
    – Word recall
    – Information speed processing

  . Frank dementia is *not* a common feature of MS.

- **Clinical evaluation**

  - Appropriate evaluation and management of depression, sleep abnormalities, pain, and fatigue should be performed in all patients with MS before formal evaluation for cognitive impairment.

  - Screening can be done using the 5-minute single-digit modality test (SDMT) or the complete 15-minute battery Brief International Cognitive Assessment for Multiple Sclerosis (BICAMS).[11]

- **Management**

  - Given the lack of substantial evidence for pharmacologic treatment of cognitive impairment in MS, nonpharmacologic approaches are more common. They include:

    - Use of personal organizers including alarm clocks, reminders, diaries, and lists
    - Job accommodations when possible
    - Cognitive rehabilitation
    - Pharmacologic agents that have shown some efficacy and are frequently used in clinical practice: armodafinil, modafinil, dalfampridine, and memantine

Emotional Changes[12–15]

- **Common symptoms**

  - Depression, anxiety, and mood swings are common in patients with MS.

- **Clinical evaluation**

  - Regular screening for mood changes should be performed in all patients with MS who develop cognitive impairment.

- **Management**

  - **Drug treatment**

    - Initial treatment with a selective serotonin reuptake inhibitor (SSRI) is a reasonable option.
    - Special considerations for patients with concomitant symptoms may include:
      - **Concomitant anxiety:** escitalopram, sertraline, or fluoxetine may be used.
      - **Concomitant pain:** duloxetine may be used in patients with neuropathic pain or chronic pain syndromes.

- o **Concomitant urinary incontinence**: imipramine and desipramine may be used.
- o **Concomitant sexual dysfunction**: bupropion and duloxetine may be considered.

- **Nondrug treatment**
  - Adequate sleep
  - Relaxation techniques
  - Cognitive-behavioral therapy
  - Maintaining healthy social networks

Dizziness and Vertigo[16,17]

- **Causes**
  - When related to MS, dizziness and vertigo result from demyelination or inflammation of the vestibular pathways.

- **Clinical evaluation**
  - Regular screening for dizziness and vertigo should be performed in all patients with MS who develop cognitive impairment.
  - It is essential to rule out benign paroxysmal positional vertigo (BPPV). In this condition, calcium debris is present within a semicircular canal; the resulting vertigo may mistakenly be attributed to MS.

- **Management**
  - There is no specific pharmacotherapy for MS-related vertigo.
  - Symptomatic relief may be beneficial and includes the use of antihistamines such as meclizine or diphenhydramine.

Dysphagia[18,19]

- **Clinical features**
  - Dysphagia is more common in advanced stages of MS but can occur at any point during the disease.
  - Both chewing and swallowing may be affected, and patients may experience choking while eating or drinking.

- **Complications**
  - When severe, dysphagia may lead to pulmonary aspiration or complete airway obstruction.

- **Clinical evaluation**

  . Regular screening for swallowing problems should be performed in all patients with MS who develop cognitive impairment.

  . A modified barium swallow test can be used to determine the severity of the symptoms and/or the need for feeding tube placement.

- **Management**

  . Depending on the severity, dietary changes may be made following evaluation by a speech/language pathologist. In some cases, tube feeding may be required.

Fatigue[20–23]

- **Clinical features**

  . Fatigue is one of the most common symptoms in patients with MS, occurring in about 80% of affected individuals.

  . It is typically described as physical exhaustion unrelated to the amount of activity performed.

  . Common features include:

    – Occurrence early in the morning despite a restful night's sleep
    – Worsening as the day progresses
    – May come on suddenly and easily
    – More severe than "normal" fatigue
    – Likely to interfere with daily responsibilities

- **Complications**

  . The cause of fatigue is currently unknown, but it is one of the primary causes of early departure from the workforce and a major contributor to overall deconditioning.

- **Clinical evaluation**

  . Regular screening for fatigue and vertigo should be performed in all patients with MS who develop cognitive impairment.

- **Management**

  . Modafinil and armodafinil are agents that promote wakefulness and are used to treat narcolepsy and obstructive sleep apnea, but have shown some efficacy in treating fatigue in patients with MS.

  . Amantadine may also be used, but has less supportive evidence in patients with MS.

. Stimulants such as methylphenidate and dextroamphetamine can also be used, keeping in mind their potential for abuse and dependence.

. **Nondrug treatment**

 – Regular physical activity to prevent deconditioning
 – Physical and occupational therapy
 – Sleep regulation
 – Stress management and relaxation training

Gait Problems[24,25]

- **Clinical features**

 . Many patients with MS will develop gait impairment, especially during the advanced stages of the disease, and some will eventually require a cane or a wheelchair.

 . It is important to identify the presence of other symptoms that may be contributing to gait impairment, including:

 – Spasticity
 – Fatigue
 – Weakness
 – Sensory problems
 – Vestibular dysfunction
 – Visual loss
 – Cerebellar dysfunction

- **Complications**

 . Patients with gait impairment are susceptible to falls and trauma-related injuries.

 . The inability to ambulate substantially contributes to disability and early departure from the workforce.

- **Clinical evaluation**

 . Regular screening for gait problems should be performed in all patients with MS who develop cognitive impairment.

- **Management**

 . Dalfampridine (4-aminopyridine) is a potassium channel blocker that can improve walking (especially walking speed) in some patients with MS.

 – Common side effects include anxiety and an increased risk for seizures.

- Physical therapy and regular strengthening exercises are important to prevent further deconditioning and progression.

Hearing Loss[26]

- **Clinical features**
  - Hearing loss is an uncommon symptom in patients with MS, but it can affect up to 6% of affected individuals. Even more rarely, hearing loss has been reported as the initial symptom of the disease.

- **Clinical evaluation**
  - Regular screening for hearing loss should be performed in all patients with MS who develop cognitive impairment.
  - Any patient with MS who experiences hearing loss should be evaluated by an audiologist.

Numbness and/or Tingling[27–30]

- **Common symptoms**
  - Patients with MS oftentimes describe diminished or altered sensation at some point during their disease.
  - The symptoms may affect one or more limbs simultaneously and may include numbness, tingling, or dysesthesias. Pain may accompany these symptoms.

- **Complications**
  - Gait difficulties may result from sensory abnormalities of the lower extremities.
  - Injuries such as burns, cuts, or other skin trauma may develop without the patient noticing and may result in infections or other complications if untreated.

- **Clinical evaluation**
  - Regular screening for sensory abnormalities should be performed in all patients with MS who develop cognitive impairment.

- **Management**
  - There are no medications to relieve sensory dysfunction. Conservative treatment and preventive strategies may help. In addition, symptomatic treatment of any associated complications should be pursued.

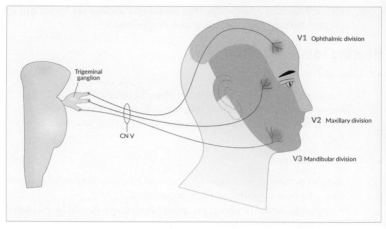

Figure 9.2 Trigeminal neuralgia pathophysiology. The trigeminal nerve (CN V) carries sensory information from the face to the brain. Inflammatory lesions may result in severe pain along any of its branches (V1, V2, V3). (A black and white version of this figure will appear in some formats. For the colour version, please refer to the plate section.)

Pain[27,31,32]

- **Clinical features**

  - Pain is a common symptom in patients with MS.
  - The specific types and severity of pain vary from patient to patient and may also change over time.
  - Pain may be described as aching, hot or burning, dull, pressure-like, squeezing, stabbing, sharp, and so forth.
  - Trigeminal neuralgia is a common complaint (Figure 9.2).

- **Clinical evaluation**

  - Regular screening for pain should be performed in all patients with MS who develop cognitive impairment.
  - It is important to assess for other possible causes of pain that are not directly related to MS, such as medication side effects, infection, trauma, and joint problems.

- **Management**

  - **Neuropathic pain**

    - This type of pain results from MS-related damage to the nerves and may range from minor discomfort to intense sharp or burning pain.

- – Anticonvulsants are some of the most commonly used medications for MS-related neuropathic pain, including carbamazepine, gabapentin, pregabalin, lamotrigine, and phenytoin. Possible side effects include skin rash, dizziness, blurred vision, and drowsiness.
- – Antidepressants are also widely used and can include tricyclic antidepressants such as amitriptyline. These agents can be useful to treat certain types of pain, such as dysesthesias. Possible side effects may include constipation, dry mouth, and blurred vision.

. **Musculoskeletal pain**

- – This type of pain originates in the muscles and joints and may result from living with the stress that MS places on the body.
  - ○ For example, balance problems or muscle weakness may lead to problems with posture that place additional strain on the joints, ligaments, or other muscles.
  - ○ Sometimes, stiffness or muscle spasms may cause pain.
- – Analgesics such as ibuprofen and other nonsteroidal anti-inflammatory drugs (NSAIDs) may be used to help control non-neuropathic pain.
- – Muscle relaxants such as baclofen, tizanidine, and cyclobenzaprine may be used. Possible side effects may include weakness, dizziness, dry mouth, and drowsiness.

. **Nondrug treatments**

- – Physical and occupational therapy
- – Regular physical activity
- – Avoiding known triggers
- – Alternative therapies such as yoga, acupuncture, meditation, and relaxation techniques

Seizures[33]

- • **Clinical features**
  - . Epilepsy is more common in patients with MS compared to the general population.
  - . Seizures in MS are generally benign and tend to respond well to treatment with antiepileptics.

- • **Clinical evaluation**
  - . Reg ular screening for seizures should be performed in all patients with MS who develop cognitive impairment.

- **Management**
  - . Antiepileptic drugs

Sexual Dysfunction[33]

- **Common symptoms**
  - . Sexual dysfunction is a common complication in patients with multiple sclerosis. Possible symptoms may include:
    - – Decreased libido
    - – Decreased arousal
    - – Anorgasmia in women
    - – Increased ejaculation latency and erectile dysfunction in men

- **Complications**
  - . All patients with sexual dysfunction should be screened for depression and use of SSRIs.

- **Clinical evaluation**
  - . Regular screening for sexual dysfunction should be performed in all patients with MS who develop cognitive impairment.

- **Management**
  - . Adequate control of neuropathic pain and spasticity, if present, may affect sexual performance in both genders. Thus, it is important to address this issue.
  - . Phosphodiesterase-5 inhibitors, such as sildenafil, are effective for the treatment of erectile dysfunction in men.
  - . Symptomatic management for complaints of vaginal dryness can be managed by regular use of vaginal lubricants during sexual intercourse.

Spasticity[5,31,34–36]

- **Clinical features**
  - . Spasticity is a common symptom in MS and refers to muscle stiffness and spasms.
  - . It results from MS-related nerve damage and causes an increase in muscle tone when the muscles are moved, creating more resistance to movement than would normally occur.
  - . Depending on the muscles affected, spasticity may make it difficult to perform delicate movements with the hands and fingers, or make larger movements difficult, including walking.

- Sometimes spasticity may cause particular problems at night.
- Triggers in some patients may include:
  - Increase in body temperature
  - Infection or disease
  - Constipation
  - A full bladder
  - Tight clothing
  - Emotional stress
  - Sudden movements

- **Complications**

  - When it affects the lower extremities, spasticity may result in significant gait impairment.
  - However, a certain amount of stiffness can help some patients keep their legs rigid and stable for walking and standing.
    - If this might be the case, close monitoring of the symptoms may be best to prevent further complications. Removing the stiffness completely may "reveal" leg weakness that may make walking much more difficult.

  - **Contractures** may develop after months or years of severe spasticity as a result of lack of muscle movement, as a joint becomes "locked" or immobilized.
    - Contractures are very difficult to treat and may lead to permanent disability.

  - **Pressure sores** may occur in the skin when patients with MS become unable to shift their own weight while sitting or lying down in bed.
    - These sores may lead to serious infections if untreated and may make spasticity worse.

- **Clinical evaluation**

  - Regular screening for spasticity should be performed in all patients with MS who develop cognitive impairment.

- **Management**

  - **Muscle relaxants**
    - This group of drugs include medications such as baclofen, tizanidine, and cyclobenzaprine. Possible side effects may include weakness, dizziness, dry mouth, and drowsiness.

- **Benzodiazepines**
  - Diazepam and clonazepam may help reduce spasticity. Side effects include drowsiness and a high potential for dependence and abuse. For this reason, these drugs are not commonly used as first-line therapy.

- **Baclofen pump**
  - This surgically implanted pump provides a continuous supply of baclofen intrathecally. When other oral treatments fail, this may be an option for some patients.

- **Cannabinoids**
  - Cannabinoids are thought to help alleviate spasticity in MS but there is no evidence to support their use from large controlled clinical trials.
  - Side effects may include confusion, sedation, and dry mouth.
  - These agents are not used as first-line therapy, and laws and regulations regarding their use differ from region to region.

- **Nondrug treatments**
  - Physical therapy
  - Occupational therapy
  - Orthotics

Speech Problems[5,36]

- **Clinical features**
  - Brainstem dysfunction may lead to dysarthria in some patients, especially in those with advanced MS.

- **Complications**
  - These symptoms may increase a patient's risk for aspiration, infection, and respiratory failure.

- **Clinical evaluation**
  - Regular screening for speech problems should be performed in all patients with MS who develop cognitive impairment.
  - All patients with speech problems should be evaluated by a speech/ language pathologist. Swallowing function should also be assessed.

- **Management**
  - Speech therapy is the mainstay of treatment for dysarthria.

. When/if present, dysphagia should be treated appropriately (see the Dysphagia section).

Tremor[37,38]

- **Clinical features**

    . Tremor in patients with MS may vary in severity and intensity.

    . MS-related tremor is typically typically caused by demyelination in the cerebellum, but brain and brainstem lesions may also cause tremors.

    . **Intention tremor**

        – This type of tremor occurs during physical movement of a limb and is not present at rest.

        – It is both the most disabling form of tremor and the most common type in patients with MS.

    . **Postural tremor**

        – This type of tremor most commonly occurs while standing or sitting, but not while lying down.

    . **Resting tremor**

        – This type of tremor is most pronounced while at rest and is more typical of Parkinson's disease than of MS.

- **Complications**

    . Tremor may make some activities of daily living challenging, such as dressing, eating, drinking, and driving.

    . It can have a significant emotional and social impact on some patients.

- **Clinical evaluation**

    . Regular screening for tremor should be performed in all patients with MS who develop cognitive impairment.

    . Familial tremor, exaggerated physiological tremor, or tremor due to a medication side effect should be ruled out in all patients with MS who develop a tremor.

- **Management**

    . **Drug management**

        – There are no approved medications for the treatment of tremor. Some agents may be used off-label but may be associated with unpleasant side effects. These include:

- ○ Beta-blockers, such as propranolol
- ○ Anticonvulsants, such as gabapentin
- ○ Benzodiazepines, such as clonazepam
- ○ Botulinum toxin

. **Surgical intervention**

- – In some cases, thalamotomy or deep brain stimulation (DBS) may be performed, but this is not commonly done.

. **Nondrug interventions**

- – Physical therapy
- – Occupational therapy
- – Lifestyle changes, such as the increasing size of keyboards or using voice-activated software

Vision Problems[27,36]

- **Clinical features**

  . **Optic neuritis** may cause transient visual loss as a result of an MS relapse, and in some cases may result in permanent visual deficits.

  - – Pain with eye movement is usually a feature of optic neuritis.
  - – Color vision may be affected.

  . **Diplopia** may occur when there is damage to one of the brainstem nuclei of cranial nerves III, IV, or VI.
  . **Nystagmus** may also occur in some patients. When severe, it may result in significant disability.

- **Clinical evaluation**

  . Regular visual screening should be performed in all patients with MS who develop cognitive impairment.

- **Management**

  . If these symptoms are the result of an MS relapse, corticosteroid treatment may hasten recovery in most cases.
  . No pharmacologic treatment has been proven to help chronic neurologic dysfunction.
  . Patching one eye in patients with diplopia may help relieve some of the symptoms, especially while driving. In addition, prism lenses may be helpful.

- All patients with vision problems should be evaluated by an ophthalmologist.

Weakness[35,36,39,40]

- **Clinical features**
  - Muscle weakness can occur in any part of the body in patients with MS.

- **Complications**
  - Lack of movement will lead to deconditioning.
  - Weakness may increase feelings of fatigue and make spasticity worse.
  - Gait may be significantly affected.

- **Clinical evaluation**
  - Regular screening for weakness should be performed in all patients with MS who develop cognitive impairment.

- **Management**
  - Management of weakness is supportive and involves a combination of:
    - Physical therapy
    - Occupational therapy
    - Sleep hygiene
    - Pacing one's work
    - Taking breaks periodically

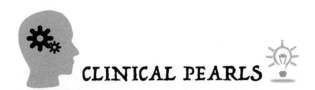

CLINICAL PEARLS

- Symptoms of MS vary considerably from person to person and change over time.
- Most of these symptoms can be alleviated, but very few can be eliminated completely.
- Not all symptoms associated with MS are directly related to inflammation of the central nervous system.

- Although treatment of the disease itself is of major importance, treatment of secondary symptoms is equally important, as failure to do so can compromise quality of life for both patients and their families.
- Regular monitoring of MS-associated symptoms is recommended. Nondrug therapies should be incorporated as adjuvants to pharmacologic treatment.

References

1. Yang CC. Bladder management in multiple sclerosis. *Phys Med Rehabil Clin North Am.* 2013;24(4):673–86. https://doi.org/10.1016/j.pmr.2013.06.004

2. Fowler CJ, Panicker JN, Drake M, et al. A UK consensus on the management of the bladder in multiple sclerosis. *J Neurol Neurosurg Psychiatry.* 2009;80(5):470–7. doi:10.1136/jnnp.2008.159178

3. Kragt JJ, Hoogervorst ELJ, Uitdehaag BMJ, Polman CH. Relation between objective and subjective measures of bladder dysfunction in multiple sclerosis. *Neurology.* 2004;63(9):1716–8. doi:10.1212/01.WNL.0000143062.43325.C8

4. Chataway J, Schuerer N, Alsanousi A, et al. Effect of high-dose simvastatin on brain atrophy and disability in secondary progressive multiple sclerosis (MS-STAT): a randomised, placebo-controlled, Phase 2 trial. *Lancet.* 2014;383(9936):2213–21. doi:10.1016/S0140-6736(13)62242-4

5. Frohman TC, Castro W, Shah A, et al. Symptomatic therapy in multiple sclerosis. *Ther Adv Neurol Disord.* 2011;4(2):83–98. doi:10.1177/1756285611400658

6. DasGupta R, Fowler CJ. Bladder, bowel and sexual dysfunction in multiple sclerosis. *Drugs.* 2003;63(2):153–66. doi:10.2165/00003495-200363020-00003

7. Rosti-Otajärvi EM, Hämäläinen PI. Neuropsychological rehabilitation for multiple sclerosis. *Cochrane Database Syst Rev.* 2014;(2). doi:10.1002/14651858.CD009131. pub3

8. Krupp LB, Christodoulou C, Melville P, et al. Donepezil improved memory in multiple sclerosis in a randomized clinical trial. *Neurology.* 2004;63(9):1579–85. doi:10.1212/01.WNL.0000142989.09633.5A

9. Patti F. Treatment of cognitive impairment in patients with multiple sclerosis. *Expert Opin Investig Drugs.* 2012;21(11):1679–99. doi:10.1517/13543784.2012.716036

10. He D, Zhang Y, Dong S, et al. Pharmacological treatment for memory disorder in multiple sclerosis. *Cochrane Database Syst Rev.* 2013;(12). doi:10.1002/14651858.CD008876.pub3

11. Langdon DW, Amato MP, Boringa J, et al. Recommendations for a brief international cognitive assessment for multiple sclerosis (BICAMS). *Mult Scler.* 2012;18(6):891–8.

12. Feinstein A. Multiple sclerosis, disease modifying treatments and depression: a critical methodological review. *Mult Scler J*. 2000;6(5):343–48. doi:10.1177/135245850000600509

13. Geraldes R, Ciccarelli O, Barkhof F, et al. The current role of MRI in differentiating multiple sclerosis from its imaging mimics. *Nat Rev Neurol*. 2018;14(4):199–213. doi:10.1038/nrneurol.2018.14

14. Sati P, Oh J, Todd Constable R, et al. The central vein sign and its clinical evaluation for the diagnosis of multiple sclerosis: a consensus statement from the North American Imaging in Multiple Sclerosis Cooperative. *Nat Rev Neurol*. 2016;12 (12):714–22. doi:10.1038/nrneurol.2016.166

15. Kearney H, Miller DH, Ciccarelli O. Spinal cord MRI in multiple sclerosis: diagnostic, prognostic and clinical value. *Nat Rev Neurol*. 2015;11(6):327–38. doi:10.1038/nrneurol.2015.80

16. Baloh RW. Vestibular neuritis. *N Engl J Med*. 2003;348(11):1027–32. doi:10.1056/NEJMcp021154

17. Kish T. Promising multiple sclerosis agents in late-stage development. *PT*. 2018;43(12):750–72. www.ncbi.nlm.nih.gov/pubmed/30559588

18. Tzelepis GE, McCool FD. Respiratory dysfunction in multiple sclerosis. *Respir Med*. 2015;109(6):671–9. doi:10.1016/j.rmed.2015.01.018

19. Yan Y, Li Y, Fu Y, et al. Autoantibody to MOG suggests two distinct clinical subtypes of NMOSD. *Sci China Life Sci*. 2016;59(12):1270–81. doi:10.1007/s11427-015-4997-y

20. Neuteboom R, Wilbur C, Van Pelt D, et al. The spectrum of inflammatory acquired demyelinating syndromes in children. *Semin Pediatr Neurol*. 2017;24(3):189–200. doi:10.1016/j.spen.2017.08.007

21. Sands MJ, Levitin A. Basics of magnetic resonance imaging. *Semin Vasc Surg*. 2004;17(2):66–82. doi:10.1053/j.semvascsurg.2004.03.011

22. Radue EW, Bendfeldt K, Mueller-Lenke N, et al. Brain atrophy: an in-vivo measure of disease activity in multiple sclerosis. *Swiss Med Wkly*. 2013;143:1–11. doi:10.4414/smw.2013.13887

23. Pucci E, Branãs P, D'Amico R, et al. Amantadine for fatigue in multiple sclerosis. *Cochrane Database Syst Rev*. 2007;2007(1):CD002818. doi:10.1002/14651858.CD002818.pub2

24. Barrett CL, Mann GE, Taylor PN, Strike P. A randomized trial to investigate the effects of functional electrical stimulation and therapeutic exercise on walking performance for people with multiple sclerosis. *Mult Scler J*. 2009;15(4):493–504. doi:10.1177/1352458508101320

25. Goodman AD, Brown TR, Krupp LB, et al. Sustained-release oral fampridine in multiple sclerosis: a randomised, double-blind, controlled trial. *Lancet*. 2009;373(9665):732–8. doi:10.1016/S0140-6736(09)60442-6

26. Fischer C, Mauguière F, Ibanez V, et al. The acute deafness of definite multiple sclerosis: BAEP patterns. *Electroencephalogr Clin Neurophysiol.* 1985;61(1):7–15. doi:10.1016/0013-4694(85)91066-1

27. Gelfand JM. *Multiple Sclerosis: Diagnosis, Differential Diagnosis, and Clinical Presentation.* Vol 122. Goodin DS, ed. Amsterdam: Elsevier; 2014. doi:10.1016/B978-0-444-52001-2.00011-X.

28. Eriksson M, Andersen O, Runmarker B. Long-term follow up of patients with clinically isolated syndromes, relapsing-remitting and secondary progressive multiple sclerosis. *Mult Scler.* 2003;9:260–74.

29. Scalfari A, Neuhaus A, Daumer M, et al. Early relapses, onset of progression, and late outcome in multiple sclerosis. *JAMA Neurol.* 2013;70(2):214–22. doi:10.1001/jamaneurol.2013.599

30. Olek MJ. Differential diagnosis, clinical features, and prognosis of multiple sclerosis. *Curr Clin Neurol Mult Scler.* 2005:15–53.

31. Willis MA, Fox RJ. Progressive multiple sclerosis. *Continuum (Minneap Minn).* 2016;22(3):785–98. doi:10.1007/978-1-4471-2395-8

32. Wingerchuk DM, Carter JL. Multiple sclerosis: current and emerging disease-modifying therapies and treatment strategies. *Mayo Clin Proc.* 2014;89(2):225–40. doi:10.1016/j.mayocp.2013.11.002

33. Nyquist PA, Cascino GD, Rodriguez M. Seizures in patients with multiple sclerosis seen at Mayo Clinic, Rochester, Minn, 1990–1998. *Mayo Clin Proc.* 2001;76 (10):983-986. doi:10.4065/76.10.983

34. Sarioglu B, Serdaroglu G, Tutuncuoglu S, Ozer EA. The use of botulinum toxin type A treatment in children with spasticity. *Pediatr Neurol.* 2003;29(4):299–301. doi:10.1016/S0887-8994(03)00269-8

35. Feinstein A, Freeman J, Lo AC. Treatment of progressive multiple sclerosis: what works, what does not, and what is needed. *Lancet Neurol.* 2015;14(2):194–207.

36. Coyle PK. Symptom management and lifestyle modifications in multiple sclerosis. *Continuum (Minneap Minn).* 2016;22(3):815–36. doi:10.1212/CON.0000000000000325

37. Tornes L, Conway B, Sheremata W. Multiple sclerosis and the cerebellum. *Neurol Clin.* 2014;32:957–77.

38. Ingram G, Hirst CL, Robertson NP. What is the risk of permanent disability from a multiple sclerosis relapse? *Neurology.* 2010;75(9):837.

39. Ching B, Mohamed A, Khoo T, Ismail H. Multiphasic disseminated encephalomyelitis followed by optic neuritis in a child with gluten sensitivity. *Mult Scler J.* 2015;21(9):1209–11. doi:10.1177/

40. Freedman MS, Rush CA. Severe, highly active, or aggressive multiple sclerosis. *Continuum (Minneap Minn).* 2016;22(3):761–84. doi:10.1212/CON.0000000000000331

Chapter 10

Reproductive Issues
Andrew Smith, MD

Introduction

With multiple sclerosis (MS) affecting women two to three times more often than men, and an average age of onset of 20–50 years, a good portion of MS patients will be women of reproductive potential. Therefore, it is critical to develop an understanding of how the disease affects reproduction and menopause, and how it might impact their life goals. Over the course of this chapter, epidemiological risk factors based on gender, pregnancy, and the need for family planning will be reviewed.

Sex, the Immune System, and Multiple Sclerosis

- Gender plays an important role in the risk of developing MS and the accumulation of disability.
- The sex ratio:[1]
  . In the 19402, the women-to mcn sex ratio was estimated to be 1:1.
  . Over the next 50 years, this ratio increased to about 2–3.5:1.
    – This was perhaps due to an increase in prevalence of relapsing-remitting MS (RRMS) in women.
    – The prevalence in men remains unchanged.
  . The sex ratio incidence rate reaches its maximum shortly after puberty and reaches unity around the of age of 59 years.

Hormones

- Differences in sex hormones and chromosomes play a major role in the increased incidence of RRMS in women.
  . The relatively low levels of estrogen in nonpregnant menstruating women favor an immune-intolerant state.

- This leads to a greater risk of autoimmune disease in women in general compared to men.

. Testosterone and pregnancy levels of estrogen typically favor a more immunotolerant state that is protective against most autoimmune diseases.

- Small studies have demonstrated a benefit of estrogen therapy on magnetic resonance imaging (MRI) outcomes in women with MS.[2]

Genetics

- In women, the presence of two X chromosomes inherently increases the strength of the immune response for two reasons:

  . **Lyonization.** Either the maternal or paternal X chromosome is permanently and randomly inactivated early on in embryological development.
  . **Parental imprinting.** Genes are expressed differently depending on the parental origin.

    - An example is the *Forkhead box p3* (*Foxp3*) gene located on the X chromosome.
      ○ This transcription factor controls T regulator (Treg) function and development.
      ○ *Fox3p* of paternal origin is not activated.[3]
      ○ Consequently, about half of women's T regulatory cells are less functional, making their immune system less tolerant and more likely to develop autoimmune disease.

- In addition to the X chromosome, other genetic factors increase women's susceptibility to MS.

  . The HLA-DR allele within the major histocompatibility complex (MHC) on chromosome 6 has been associated with the risk of MS.

    - Women are at higher risk of receiving the HLA-DRB1 allele through disproportionate maternal transmission from their mother.[5]

Epigenetics and Environmental Factors

- The increased rate of MS in women over the last 50 years is thought to be due to an underlying epigenetic phenomenon.
- Several factors have changed over this period of time, including:

- Increases in adiposity of the general population.

  - Higher rates of obesity in young women, in particular, appear to increase the rates of MS.

- Decreasing age of menarche.[6]

  - This may be a consequence of increased obesity rates.
  - Younger age at menarche is associated with an increased risk of developing MS.[7,8]
    - This may be due to an increase in the amount of time spent in a low-estrogen state.[9]

- Another potential risk factor for women is having children at a later age.[10]

  - Studies have shown that women who become pregnant at a younger age have a decreased risk of developing MS compared to those who become pregnant later in life.
    - Pregnancy appears to provide protection against the risk of developing MS by shifting the immune system away from the highly immunogenic T1 response, presumably due to high estrogen levels during pregnancy.
  - Other factors of Westernization:
    - Decreased exposure to sunlight
    - Increased rate of smoking in women[11,12]

Family Planning

Family planning is a critical, yet often overlooked part of MS care. Evidence suggests that a patient's lack of critical knowledge regarding MS care could affect his or her decision about having children.

Oral Contraceptives

- The data surrounding the use of oral contraceptives (OCPs) in women with MS are mixed.

  - Some studies suggest that birth control use may increase the risk of developing MS (or MS-related attacks) due to the delay in time before the first pregnancy.[13]
  - Others suggest that OCPs do not increase the risk of developing MS or of accumulating disease-related disability, and that they may even reduce the risk of developing MS in the short term.[14]

- Population-based studies have shown that the rate of MS is significantly reduced in women who take OCPs.[15]
- Data on the long-term use of oral contraceptives in women with MS suggest that birth control pills are associated with less disability over the disease course.[16,17]

- In general, the efficacy of OCPs does not appear to be compromised or affected by the use of disease-modifying therapies (DMTs).
- However, OCPs may interact with many of the medications used as symptomatic treatments in MS.

  - Always review all medications a patient takes and consider their effects on birth control to limit the risk of unintended pregnancies.

Fertility and Multiple Sclerosis

- Despite the fact that MS does not generally affect fertility, approximately 80% of women choose not to become pregnant following diagnosis.

  - Of these, about one-third base their decision on the diagnosis itself.[18–20]
  - Further exacerbating the problem, sexual dysfunction can be significant in these women and can affect their desire and ability to conceive.

Assistive Reproductive Techniques

- Women with MS are more likely to use assistive reproductive techniques (ART) in an effort to conceive. This can lead to:

  - A seven-fold increase in MS relapse rates
  - A nine-fold increase in MRI activity[21]

- While the use of either gonadotropin-releasing hormone (GnRH) agonists or antagonists can lead to an increased rate of relapse, the risk appears to be higher with GnRH agonists.[21–23]
- One strategy to reduce this risk involves treatment with high-dose corticosteroids after every unsuccessful menstrual cycle in women who are actively trying to conceive.[24–28]

Multiple Sclerosis and Pregnancy

- Until the PRegnancy in MS Study (PRIMS) trial was completed, women with MS were generally discouraged from having children.
- The PRIMS study demonstrated that pregnancy had a net neutral effect on disease activity.

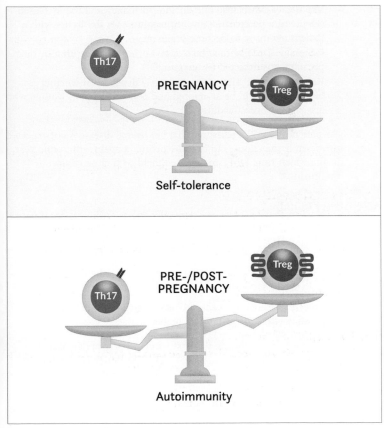

Figure 10.1 Effect of pregnancy on autoimmune disease. In general, a state of self-tolerance and reduced autoimmune activity can be expected during pregnancy, characterized by a shift toward a more anti-inflammatory milieu via T regulatory cell (Treg) activity and away from Th17-mediated inflammation. The opposite is true in the pre- or post-pregnancy period.

- A decrease in relapse rates during each trimester in pregnant women can be expected.
- However, a relapse "rebound" may follow within the first three months post-delivery (Figure 10.1).

- – The decreased relapse rate during pregnancy and the increased relapse rate postpartum are important issues to discuss with a patient planning to become pregnant.
- – Generally, DMT should be stopped prior to conception or once pregnancy is detected (if unexpected).
- – Restarting DMT after delivery largely depends on whether breastfeeding will be attempted and is not advised in women who are actively breastfeeding.

- . The patient should be reassured that her overall disease is not expected to worsen if she chooses to become pregnant again within one year, during which time DMT may be withheld with close clinical monitoring.[26]

Relapse in Pregnancy

- Fortunately, MS relapses during pregnancy are relatively rare.[27–38]
- In the case of a relapse during pregnancy, consideration may be given to treating these relapses like any other exacerbation (see Chapter 1).

  - . If needed, a short course of corticosteroids after the first trimester is generally considered safe.

    - – Careful consideration should also be given to this treatment's possible effect on gestational diabetes.

  - . The use of steroids during the first trimester is generally not recommended due to an increased risk of birth defects, such as cleft palate.

- Due to the decreased rate of relapse during pregnancy, it is commonly believed that the average patient with MS does not require DMT during pregnancy.

  - . There are always exceptions to this rule, however. This decision should be made only under the care of an MS specialist on a case-by-case basis.

- It is important to understand the consequences of discontinuing highly effective therapy and the associated risks of rebound disease during and after pregnancy.

  - . Rebound disease is defined as more aggressive or severe attacks that occur after discontinuing highly effective DMTs.
  - . Treatment of rebound disease generally consists of reinitiation of the patient's pre-pregnancy DMT.

- Alternatively, other methods may be used to control the rebound disease such as pulse steroids or intravenous immunoglobulin (IVIG).

- Some evidence suggests that pregnancy may have a long-term benefit on the disease course of patients with MS.

  - Women who became pregnant at least two times following a diagnosis of MS have been noted to reach disability milestones at a later age than those who were never pregnant.[37]

Delivery

- Except for very disabled patients, MS appears to have a minimal effect on delivery.
- Obstetricians should treat their patients with MS like any other patients, but communication with the treating neurologist is always recommended.
- The use of spinal anesthesia, epidural anesthesia, or no anesthesia during labor does not appear to increase the risk of disability progression or postpartum relapse in women with MS.
- Population-based studies suggest that MS does not necessarily increase the need for labor induction or augmentation.[37]

Breastfeeding

- Currently available data on breastfeeding by women with MS are mostly in favor of this practice.

  - Breastfeeding does not appear to increase the risk of postpartum relapse in women with MS.
  - Several studies suggest that exclusive breastfeeding may be protective from a relapse in the postpartum period.
  - Breastfeeding should be discouraged only in patients with aggressive disease so that they can resume highly efficacious therapy.[31]
  - In women with MS who wish to breastfeed and to resume DMT, consideration may be given to the use of glatiramer acetate and the interferons during this time.

    - Both of these therapies consist of large molecules that are not orally available and have a low chance of being present in breast milk.[27,32]

- During breastfeeding:

  - If the patient requires high-dose steroid treatment due to a relapse, it is typically recommended to "pump and dump" for at least 4–6 hours after the infusion.[32]

– To be safe, it is common practice to recommend "pumping and dumping" for 12 to 24 hours after an MRI with gadolinium contrast.[34] After this time, breastfeeding may be resumed.

Disease-Modifying Therapy Use in Pregnancy

While this section reviews the potential use of DMTs, it is important to note that none of these medications has FDA approval for use during pregnancy.

- DMTs should be discontinued when attempts to conceive are initiated.
- It is generally recommended to discontinue DMT at least five half-lives prior to the initial attempt at conception.

This section reviews available data on "washout" procedures for DMT use during pregnancy. It is important to note that continued use of DMT in pregnancy should occur only under the supervision of an experienced MS specialist.

Injectable Therapies

Overall, the injectable therapies have the longest-term safety data on pregnancy exposure of any DMTs.

- **Glatiramer acetate**
  - This agent is currently considered the safest DMT in women of childbearing potential.
  - It is not FDA-approved for use in pregnancy, but the European Medicines Agency (EMA) removed its restriction on use during pregnancy in 2016.
  - Pregnancy registry data in more than 7,400 patients over a 20-year span have demonstrated no increased risk of congenital birth defects or abortions.[35]
  - Therefore, glatiramer acetate could arguably be continued throughout the entire course of the pregnancy if deemed necessary.

- **Interferons**
  - Interferons are second to glatiramer acetate regarding the amount of information known about their risks during pregnancy.
  - They can generally be considered the next safest agents for use during pregnancy.
    - Early data from pregnancies exposed to interferons demonstrated a lower mean birth weight, shorter birth length, higher rate of abortion, and higher rate of premature births.

- However, more recent data from larger pregnancy registries did not identify any risks from early exposure to interferons during the first trimester.[36]

Oral Therapies

- A "washout" period is recommended in all patients taking these medications before they attempt to become pregnant.
- Unlike the injectables and monoclonal antibody infusions, oral therapies consist of small molecules that can cross the placenta before the patient becomes aware of the pregnancy.
- Fingolimod is associated with an increased risk of cardiac defects. In contrast, there is no evidence of such a risk in humans exposed to either teriflunomide or dimethyl fumarate.[36]

  - However, the number of human pregnancies exposed to these agents is very low, and they have been shown to have some teratogenic potential in animal models. Thus, a potential for teratogenicity in humans may exist.
  - It is important to discuss family planning with patients who have MS prior to the initiation of any of these agents.[37]

- **Fingolimod**

  - Fingolimod has a half-life of 6–9 days, and the recommended washout period prior to conception is 2 months.[38]

    - An important consideration during the washout period is the risk of severe rebound disease.
    - Roughly one-third of patients will have a relapse during pregnancy upon discontinuation of fingolimod.[39]
    - These risks should be reviewed with the patient prior to starting or discontinuing fingolimod.

- **Dimethyl fumarate**

  - Dimethyl fumarate's half-life is on the order of hours.
  - The drug is typically cleared within 24 hours from the system after the last ingestion.
  - Although the typically recommended washout period is 1 month, it could be shorter.

- **Teriflunomide**

  - The half-life of this medication is approximately 18–19 days.

- The drug may remain detectable for up to 2 years after discontinuation.
- Consequently, patients must undergo a rapid elimination protocol with either cholestyramine at doses of 4–8 g every 8 hours for 11 days or activated charcoal at doses of 50 g every 12 hours for 11 days.[40]
- Because teriflunomide can be found in semen, it is recommended that men undergo a rapid elimination protocol prior to attempting to conceive.

  – This recommendation is not found on the European label.[41]

Infusion Therapies

- With the exception of natalizumab, infusion therapies are newer agents with more limited data regarding their use in women of childbearing potential.
- Infusion therapies are generally considered very highly efficacious, and significant planning is required prior to their discontinuation for a planned conception, keeping in mind that rebound disease is possible.
- **Natalizumab**

  - Natalizumab was the first highly efficacious therapy to receive approval for use in patients with MS.
  - Since it is a large molecule, it is not expected to cross the placenta. This drug is typically eliminated from the body within 2 months after the last dose.

    – Consequently, some providers advocate for the use of this medication until the time of conception.[42]

  - Data from the natalizumab pregnancy registry suggest that there may be an increased risk of birth defects with use of this medication.[43]

    – However, no specific patterns of birth defects have been identified.[44]
    – Although only limited data on this strategy are available, it should be noted that there is a risk of hematological abnormalities in the offspring of those women who receive natalizumab during the third trimester.[45]

- **Alemtuzumab**

  - Alemtuzumab is somewhat unique in its ability to provide a durable effect without the need for constant retreatment.[46]

- About half of patients who receive alemtuzumab will not require retreatment for about an 8-year period.
  - This medication can provide a potential long window during which a woman could attempt to conceive and be protected from MS relapses while not actively on a DMT.
  - The formal washout recommendation is 4 months after the last infusion.
  - Therefore, in patients with aggressive disease who can wait 16 months to attempt conception, alemtuzumab becomes a potential treatment option.
- One special consideration to review with the patient is the potential risk of developing additional autoimmune diseases.
  - Fetal transfer of antibodies secondary to autoimmune conditions has also been reported.[32]

- **Anti-CD20 monoclonal agents (rituximab and ocrelizumab)**
  - The formally recommended washout periods for these drugs are 12 and 6 months, respectively.
  - These agents are also an attractive option for patients considering pregnancy.
    - CD19 counts can remain suppressed for as long as 9–12 months following an infusion in some patients.
      - This could create a window of opportunity during which patients may attempt to achieve pregnancy while protection is ongoing.
    - Typically, CD19 counts are monitored beginning in the fifth month of pregnancy to estimate the time for retreatment when B-cell repletion begins.
    - Allowing for proper washout of these agents is important due to the risk of B-cell depletion and other hematological abnormalities that may affect the exposed fetus.[47]

Restarting DMT after Pregnancy

- In patients who are not planning to breastfeed, DMT may be restarted as soon as the patient has recovered from the delivery.
  - Data suggest that restarting therapy early can reduce the risk of postpartum relapses.[31]

- In those patients who are planning to breastfeed, plans should be made in advance to restart their DMT soon after breastfeeding stops.

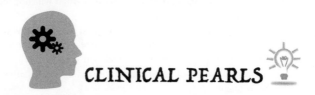

CLINICAL PEARLS

- Because MS affects women more often than men and has an average age of onset in women of 20–50 years, a good portion of MS patients will be women of reproductive potential.
- Although there are no guidelines specifying when to stop DMT prior to conception, family planning is a critical part of MS care.
- None of the DMTs are approved for use during pregnancy, and it is recommended to discontinue DMTs at least five half-lives prior to the initial attempt at conception.
- Overall, the injectable therapies have more safety data related to pregnancy exposure compared to any of the other DMTs.
- Breastfeeding is encouraged in patients who have MS, but DMTs should be withheld until breastfeeding ends. Breastfeeding should be discouraged only in patients with aggressive disease so as to restart highly efficacious therapy.

References

1. Trojano M, Lucchese G, Graziano G, et al. Geographical variations in sex ratio trends over time in multiple sclerosis. *PLoS One*. 2012;7(10):e48078.

2. Ysrraelit MC, Correale J. Impact of sex hormones on immune function and multiple sclerosis development. *Immunology*. 2019;156(1):9–22.

3. Fontenot JD, Gavin MA, Rudensky AY. Pillars article: *Foxp3* programs the development and function of CD4+CD25+ regulatory T cells. *J Immunol*. 2017;198(3):986–92.

4. Voskuhl RR, Sawalha AH, Itoh Y. Sex chromosome contributions to sex differences in multiple sclerosis susceptibility and progression. *Mult Scler*. 2018;24(1):22–31.

5. Haines JL, Terwedow HA, Burgess K, et al. Linkage of the MHC to familial multiple sclerosis suggests genetic heterogeneity. The Multiple Sclerosis Genetics Group. *Hum Mol Genet*. 1998;7(8):1229–34.

6. Mosca L, Mantero V, Penco S, et al. HLA-DRB1*15 association with multiple sclerosis is confirmed in a multigenerational Italian family. *Funct Neurol*. 2017;32(2):83–8.

7. Biro FM, Khoury P, Morrison JA. Influence of obesity on timing of puberty. *Int J Androl.* 2006;29(1):272–7; discussion 86–90.

8. Chitnis T. Role of puberty in multiple sclerosis risk and course. *Clin Immunol.* 2013;149(2):192–200.

9. Mohammadbeigi A, Kazemitabaee M, Etemadifar M. Risk factors of early onset of MS in women in reproductive age period: survival analysis approach. *Arch Womens Ment Health.* 2016;19(4):681–6.

10. Waubant E. Effect of puberty on multiple sclerosis risk and course. *Mult Scler.* 2018;24(1):32–5.

11. Koch-Henriksen N, Sorensen PS. The changing demographic pattern of multiple sclerosis epidemiology. *Lancet Neurol.* 2010;9(5):520–32.

12. Degelman ML, Herman KM. Smoking and multiple sclerosis: a systematic review and meta-analysis using the Bradford Hill criteria for causation. *Mult Scler Relat Disord.* 2017;17:207–16.

13. Rotstein DL, Chen H, Wilton AS, et al. Temporal trends in multiple sclerosis prevalence and incidence in a large population. *Neurology.* 2018;90(16):e1435–41.

14. Hellwig K, Chen LH, Stancyzk FZ, Langer-Gould AM. Oral contraceptives and multiple sclerosis/clinically isolated syndrome susceptibility.*PLoS One.* 2016;11(3):e0149094.

15. Alonso A, Jick SS, Olek MJ, et al. Recent use of oral contraceptives and the risk of multiple sclerosis.*Arch Neurol.* 2005;62(9):1362–5.

16. Cavalla P, Rovei V, Masera S, et al. Fertility in patients with multiple sclerosis: current knowledge and future perspectives. *Neurol Sci.* 2006;27(4):231–9.

17. Gava G, Bartolomei I, Costantino A, et al. Long-term influence of combined oral contraceptive use on the clinical course of relapsing-remitting multiple sclerosis. *Fertil Steril.* 2014;102(1):116–22.

18. Sena A, Couderc R, Vasconcelos JC, et al. Oral contraceptive use and clinical outcomes in patients with multiple sclerosis. *J Neurol Sci.* 2012;317(1–2):47–51.

19. Thone J, Kollar S, Nousome D, et al. Serum anti-Mullerian hormone levels in reproductive-age women with relapsing-remitting multiple sclerosis. *Mult Scler.* 2015;21(1):41–7.

20. Ferraro D, Simone AM, Adani G, et al. Definitive childlessness in women with multiple sclerosis: a multicenter study. *Neurol Sci.* 2017;38(8):1453–9.

21. Alwan S, Yee IM, Dybalski M, et al. Reproductive decision making after the diagnosis of multiple sclerosis (MS). *Mult Scler.* 2013;19(3):351–8.

22. Correale J, Farez MF, Ysrraelit MC. Increase in multiple sclerosis activity after assisted reproduction technology. *Ann Neurol.* 2012;72(5):682–94.

23. Hellwig K, Correale J. Artificial reproductive techniques in multiple sclerosis. *Clin Immunol.* 2013;149(2):219–24.

24. Michel L, Foucher Y, Vukusic S, et al. Increased risk of multiple sclerosis relapse after in vitro fertilisation. *J Neurol Neurosurg Psychiatry.* 2012;83(8):796–802.

25. Bove R, Alwan S, Friedman JM, et al. Management of multiple sclerosis during pregnancy and the reproductive years: a systematic review. *Obstet Gynecol.* 2014;124 (6):1157–68.

26. Parnell GP, Booth DR. The multiple sclerosis (MS) genetic risk factors indicate both acquired and innate immune cell subsets contribute to MS pathogenesis and identify novel therapeutic opportunities. *Front Immunol.* 2017;8:425.

27. Confavreux C, Hutchinson M, Hours MM, et al. Rate of pregnancy-related relapse in multiple sclerosis. Pregnancy in Multiple Sclerosis Group. *N Engl J Med.* 1998;339(5):285–91.

28. D'Hooghe MB, Nagels G, Uitdehaag BM. Long-term effects of childbirth in MS. *J Neurol Neurosurg Psychiatry.* 2010;81(1):38–41.

29. Lu E, Zhu F, van der Kop M, et al. Labor induction and augmentation in women with multiple sclerosis. *Mult Scler.* 2013;19(9):1182–9.

30. Vukusic S, Durand-Dubief F, Benoit A, et al. Natalizumab for the prevention of post-partum relapses in women with multiple sclerosis. *Mult Scler.* 2015;21 (7):953–5.

31. Coyle PK. Management of women with multiple sclerosis through pregnancy and after childbirth. *Ther Adv Neurol Disord.* 2016;9(3):198–210.

32. Kubik-Huch RA, Gottstein-Aalame NM, Frenzel T, et al. Gadopentetate dimeglumine excretion into human breast milk during lactation. *Radiology.* 2000;216(2):555–8.

33 Goischke HK. Safety assessment of gadolinium-based contrast agents (GBCAs) requires consideration of long-term adverse effects in all human tissues. *Mult Scler J Exp Transl Clin.* 2017;3(2):2055217317704450.

34. Sandberg-Wollheim M, Neudorfer O, Grinspan A, et al. Pregnancy outcomes from the branded glatiramer acetate pregnancy database. *Int J MS Care.* 2018;20(1):9–14.

35. Vaughn C, Bushra A, Kolb C, Weinstock-Guttman B. An update on the use of disease-modifying therapy in pregnant patients with multiple sclerosis. *CNS Drugs.* 2018;32(2):161–78.

36. Lu E, Wang BW, Alwan S, et al. A review of safety-related pregnancy data surrounding the oral disease-modifying drugs for multiple sclerosis. *CNS Drugs.* 2014;28(2):89–94.

37. Karlsson G, Francis G, Koren G, et al. Pregnancy outcomes in the clinical development program of fingolimod in multiple sclerosis. *Neurology.* 2014;82 (8):674–80.

38. Hemat S, Vidal-Jordana A, Guger M, et al., eds. Disease activity during pregnancy after fingolimod withdrawal due to planning a pregnancy in women with multiple sclerosis. Poster session presented at the 34th annual meeting of the European Committee for Treatment and Research in Multiple Sclerosis (ECTRIMS); 2018.

39. Kieseier BC, Benamor M. Pregnancy outcomes following maternal and paternal exposure to teriflunomide during treatment for relapsing-remitting multiple sclerosis. *Neurol Ther.* 2014;3(2):133–8.

40. Genzyme S. European Public Assessment Report (EPAR) for Aubagio. 2013 [updated 2018]. www.ema.europa.eu/en/medicines/human/EPAR/aubagio.

41. Kleerekooper I, van Kempen ZLE, et al. Disease activity following pregnancy-related discontinuation of natalizumab in MS. *Neurol Neuroimmunol Neuroinflamm.* 2018;5(1):e424.

42. Friend S, Richman S, Bloomgren G, et al. Evaluation of pregnancy outcomes from the Tysabri (natalizumab) pregnancy exposure registry: a global, observational, follow-up study. *BMC Neurol.* 2016;16(1):150.

43. Ebrahimi N, Herbstritt S, Gold R, et al. Pregnancy and fetal outcomes following natalizumab exposure in pregnancy: a prospective, controlled observational study. *Mult Scler.* 2015;21(2):198–205.

44. Haghikia A, Langer-Gould A, Rellensmann G, et al. Natalizumab use during the third trimester of pregnancy. *JAMA Neurol.* 2014;71(7):891–5.

45. Coles AJ, Cohen JA, Fox EJ, et al. Alemtuzumab CARE-MS II 5-year follow-up: efficacy and safety findings. *Neurology.* 2017;89(11):1117–26.

46. Das G, Damotte V, Gelfand JM, et al. Rituximab before and during pregnancy: a systematic review, and a case series in MS and NMOSD. *Neurol Neuroimmunol Neuroinflamm.* 2018;5(3):e453.

47. Achiron A, Kishner I, Dolev M, et al. Effect of intravenous immunoglobulin treatment on pregnancy and postpartum-related relapses in multiple sclerosis. *J Neurol.* 2004;251(9):1133–7.

Chapter

11

Pediatric Multiple Sclerosis

Carlos A. Pérez, MD

Recognition and diagnosis of pediatric multiple sclerosis (MS) can be challenging given the broad differential of possible MS mimics and acquired demyelinating syndrome (ADS) phenotypes. It is not uncommon for clinicians to consider alternative diagnoses rather than MS in children with acute neurologic symptoms and white matter lesions on MRI, such as leukodystrophies, vasculopathies, mitochondrial defects, or other metabolic or inflammatory disorders. Once a diagnosis is made, the current lack of understanding regarding the safety and generalizability of use of disease-modifying therapy (DMT) in children can pose additional challenges to treating children and adolescents. In this chapter, we discuss the clinical presentation, diagnostic evaluation, and treatment approach to pediatric-onset MS, paying special attention to the areas in which pediatric disease may differ from adult-onset MS.

Clinical Features
Overview

- Like adult-onset MS, pediatric MS is characterized by recurrent episodes of central nervous system (CNS) demyelination separated in time and space.[1]
- While many features overlap with adult-onset disease, there are some characteristic features specific to pediatric MS.[1,2]
- In general, younger patients (younger than 10 years) tend to have more atypical presentations.[3]

Epidemiology

- As many as 10% of all patients with MS experience their first clinical symptom before age 18.[4]
- The mean age of diagnosis among pediatric patients is approximately 15 years.[3] Although fewer than 20% of children with MS receive a diagnosis prior to age 10, the youngest patient reported to date was only 2 years old.[3]

- In adults, MS is more commonly reported in Caucasians of northern European ancestry. However, pediatric MS is more common in African Americans in the United States, and in other ethnic populations (Caribbean, Asian, and East European) in Canada.[4]
- Before puberty, the female-to-male ratio is approximately 1:1, but it increases to 3:1 in adolescents. This suggests that hormonal changes – menarche, in particular – may play an important role in the pathogenesis of MS.[5,6]

Clinical Presentation

- At onset, more than 97% of pediatric patients have relapsing-remitting MS (RRMS). A progressive disease from onset should raise suspicion for an alternative diagnosis.[7,8]
- Children may present with forms of clinically isolated syndrome (CIS), including optic neuritis, transverse myelitis, and cerebellar, brainstem, or cerebral hemispheric lesions.[9,10]
- Other symptoms that can be seen in pediatric MS that are seen less frequently in adult-onset disease include:[1,11]
  - Encephalopathy
  - Seizures
  - Polyfocal symptoms

Risk Factors

A combination of genetic, environmental, and epigenetic factors contribute to the overall risk of developing MS in susceptible individuals (Figure 11.1).

Genetic Factors

- Certain human leukocyte antigen (HLA) genes are associated with an increased risk for MS, including three HLA haplotypes: HLA DRB1*1501, DQA1*0102, and DQB1*0602.[11,12]
- The HLA-DR15 haplotype is associated with early-onset MS.[13–15]
- The overall risk for MS in first-degree relatives and dizygotic twins is 5%. In monozygotic twins, the risk is 25%.[6,16–18]

Environmental Factors

- As in adult-onset MS, previous exposure to Epstein–Barr virus has been associated with an increased risk of demyelinating disease in children.[6]
- The prevalence of MS is greater at northern latitudes (latitude gradient).[4,19]
- Vitamin D deficiency has been demonstrated to increase the risk for developing MS.[6,20]

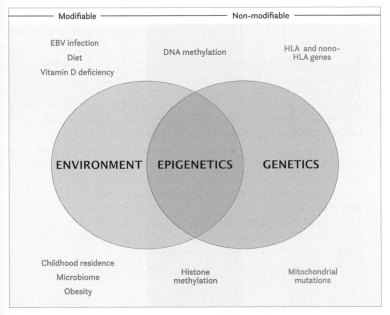

Modifiable ——————————————— Non-modifiable

EBV infection

Diet

Vitamin D deficiency

DNA methylation

HLA and nono-HLA genes

ENVIRONMENT   EPIGENETICS   GENETICS

Childhood residence

Microbiome

Obesity

Histone methylation

Mitochondrial mutations

Figure 11.1 Risk factors for the development of multiple sclerosis.

- Initial studies of gut microbiota in children with MS have shown a perturbation in the normal flora indicative of a pro-inflammatory milieu.[1,4,13,21]

Modifiable Risk Factors

- Obesity has been associated with a higher risk of developing MS.[1,13] Hence, maintaining a balanced diet and engaging in exercise are important in all children and adolescents to lower the risk of MS.
- Smoking exposure has been shown to increase the risk of MS twofold in children.[22]

Protective Factors

- Vitamin D supplementation has been shown to decrease the frequency of demyelinating relapses.
- Previous cytomegalovirus (CMV) infection has been reported to reduce the risk of MS by as much as 70%.[4,6]
- The possible role of breastfeeding as a protective factor against MS has been postulated but requires further investigation.[3,23]

Diagnostic Evaluation

Whether in the clinic or in the hospital, the goals of the first encounter with the patient and the family include:

- To arrive at a diagnosis or to develop a plan to discover the etiology of the disease
- Through history, examination, and direct observation, to obtain an accurate impression of the neurologic deficits and any other signs of emotional distress
- To establish a trusting relationship with the child or teenager and the family to facilitate appropriate, beneficial long-term treatment

Interviewing the Child/Adolescent

- After a brief introduction to the parents, the clinical should focus on the child. This is important both for diagnosis and to form a therapeutic alliance.
- An age-appropriate conversation about hobbies, sports, after-school activities, and other topics can help the child feel comfortable so that the history and examination can be more informative.
- Parents and children usually appreciate kind and direct interaction by the physician with the child.

Interviewing the Parents/Guardians

- Parents/guardians can provide the following information:
  - Verification of the details provided by the child
  - Previous episodes of neurologic deficits, diagnostic testing, and treatments
  - Academic performance
  - Detailed childhood history, including developmental history and other medical diagnoses
  - Family history of MS or other autoimmune diseases, as well as other neurologic, psychiatric, or learning disorders

- It is essential to encourage all parents to provide honest information to their child about the diagnosis. Doing so will provide the child with the opportunity to talk and ask questions during follow-up visits, as well as to share feelings and concerns.
- Diagnosing MS is especially challenging in prepubescent children due to the potential for atypical clinical and radiologic presentations in addition to the broader spectrum of possible differential diagnoses.[4]
- The International Pediatric Multiple Sclerosis Study Group (IPMSSG) published definitions for pediatric MS and related disorders most recently in 2012[24] (Table 11.1).

Table 11.1 International Pediatric Multiple Sclerosis Research Group 2012 diagnostic criteria for pediatric acute demyelinating syndromes

Clinically Isolated Syndrome (CIS)

All of the following:

- A clinical event caused by inflammatory demyelinating disease
- No previous history of similar events
- No encephalopathy except as readily explained by fever
- The criteria for a diagnosis of MS are not met on baseline magnetic resonance imaging (MRI)

Multiple Sclerosis

Any of the following:

- Two or more non-encephalopathic central nervous system (CNS) clinical events separated by more than 30 days
- Single clinical event and MRI features consistent with criteria for dissemination in space (DIS) and in which a follow-up MRI shows evidence of new lesions to fulfill criteria for dissemination in time (DIT)
- ADEM (see below) followed 3 months later by a non-encephalopathic clinical event with new lesions on brain MRI consistent with MS
- A single clinical event with MRI features consistent with criteria for both DIS and DIT

Acute Disseminated Encephalomyelitis (ADEM)

All of the following:

- A single polyfocal clinical CNS event with presumed inflammatory cause
- Encephalopathy that cannot be explained by fever is present
- MRI showing diffuse, poorly demarcated, large (1–2 cm) lesions involving predominantly the cerebral white matter; T1 hypointense white matter lesions are rare; deep gray matter lesions can be present
- No new symptoms, signs. or MRI findings after ≥3 months of the incident ADEM

Neuromyelitis Optica Spectrum Disorder (NMOSD)

All are required:

- Optic neuritis
- Acute myelitis
- At least two of the following:
- Contiguous spinal cord MRI lesions involving three or more vertebral segments
- Brain MRI not meeting diagnostic criteria for MS
- AQP4-IgG seropositive status

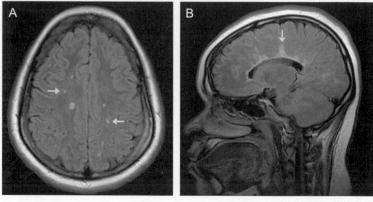

Figure 11.2 Magnetic resonance imaging (MRI) in a pediatric patient with multiple sclerosis. (A) Axial T2/FLAIR image showing white matter and juxtacortical demyelinating lesions (arrows). (B) Sagittal T2/FLAIR image showing typical Dawson's fingers (arrow).

Neuroimaging

- The typical brain magnetic resonance imaging (MRI) pattern consistent with MS in adults applies to children as well. Areas of demyelination are typically seen in the periventricular, juxtacortical, infratentorial, and spinal cord white matter[25,26] (Figure 11.2).

- In children, the factors most strongly associated with a risk of MS on initial brain MRI include:[7,27]

  - One or more T2 lesions on initial brain MRI
  - Presence of oligoclonal bands in the cerebrospinal fluid (CSF)
  - One or more hypointense T1 lesions
  - One or more periventricular lesions

- Children are more likely than adults to present with more T2 hyperintense lesions in the posterior fossa, as well as more contrast-enhancing lesions.[19,24]

  - Interestingly, these lesions are more likely to be reversible on follow-up imaging compared to those in adults, which suggests a more inflammatory disease with a chance for better recovery in children.[4]

- Although this finding is rare, some children can present with large, tumor-like demyelinating lesions on brain MRI despite only having modest neurologic deficits.[28]

- The current McDonald diagnostic criteria (see Chapter 4) may be applied to children older than age 12 if the initial presentation is not characterized by encephalopathy.[19]

Ancillary Studies

CSF Studies

- The CSF profile in children may differ from that in adults.[20]
- As many as 92% of children with MS have unmatched oligoclonal bands in CSF compared with serum, but the overall percentage may be lower in the younger age groups (younger than 12 years).[4]
- The presence of pleocytosis can be more variable and less consistent, and has been reported in 33–73% of children with MS.[6]
- As many as one-third of children with MS can have an elevated immunoglobulin G (IgG) index.[20]

Evoked Potentials

- In adults, visual evoked potentials (EPs) provide supportive evidence of demyelination in the optic nerve, brainstem, or spinal cord.[4]
- Abnormal findings can be found in as many as 95% of children with a history of optic neuritis and in as many as 60% of children with MS and no known history of optic nerve dysfunction.[4]

Differential Diagnosis

An important step in the diagnosis of children is to differentiate MS from other ADS phenotypes (Figure 11.3). About one-third of children with an ADS will be diagnosed with relapsing disease such as MS or neuromyelitis optica spectrum disorder (NMOSD)[19,29] (Figure 11.4).

Acute Disseminated Encephalomyelitis

- In children, polyfocal neurologic deficits and encephalopathy are most indicative of acute disseminated encephalomyelitis (ADEM), especially in the presence of diffuse, asymmetric, and poorly demarcated lesions on brain MRI.[1,3]
- Approximately 20% of children with ADEM will experience future relapses that meet the diagnostic criteria for MS.[17]
- Any recurrence or worsening of symptoms within 90 days of onset is considered part of the first ADEM attack.[27]
- Recurrent episodes beyond the first 90 days likely suggest recurrent demyelinating disease, and immunosuppression should probably be considered in these cases.[27]

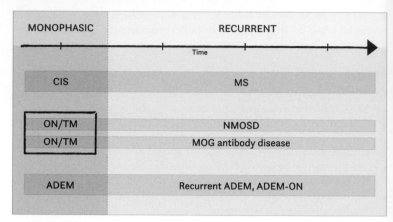

Figure 11.3 Spectrum of demyelinating diseases. Abbreviations: ADEM, acute disseminated encephalomyelitis; CIS, clinically isolated syndrome; MOG, myelin oligodendrocyte glycoprotein; MS, multiple sclerosis; NMOSD, neuromyelitis optica spectrum disorder; ON, optic neuritis; TM, transverse myelitis.

Neuromyelitis Optica Spectrum Disorder

- Neuromyelitis optica spectrum disorder (NMOSD) has been reported in children as young as 23 months.[24]
- Although it may present similarly to MS, NMOSD can be distinguished with anti-aquaporin 4 (anti-AQP4) antibody testing.[1,20]
- If initial anti-AQP4 testing is negative in children, repeat testing is recommended after 6 months.[1]
- Excluding this diagnosis is essential, as NMOSD may be worsened by MS therapies.[30]

Myelin Oligodendrocyte Glycoprotein Antibody–Associated Disease

- Serum anti–myelin oligodendrocyte glycoprotein (MOG) antibodies are present in as many as 50% of children with an ADS.[9,31]
- Unlike with children with pediatric MS, younger children (younger than 10 years) with MOG-associated disease typically present with longitudinally extensive transverse myelitis (LETM) and large, poorly demarcated ADEM-like brain lesions, while older children typically present with optic neuritis and short myelitis[19,26] (Figure 11.5).

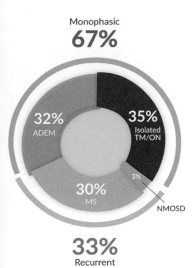

Monophasic
67%

32%
ADEM

35%
Isolated
TM/ON

30%
MS

3%
NMOSD

33%
Recurrent

Figure 11.4 Acute demyelinating syndromes in children. Abbreviations: ADEM, acute disseminated encephalomyelitis; MS, multiple sclerosis; NMOSD, neuromyelitis optica spectrum disorder; ON, optic neuritis; TM, transverse myelitis.

- The older pediatric group (older than 10 years) has been shown to have an increased risk for recurrent disease, and some of these patients will eventually receive a diagnosis of MS.[26]

Other Disorders

- In children with nonspecific CSF abnormalities and abnormal MRI with evidence of white matter lesions, other conditions should be considered, including:[4,17,22]
  - Neoplastic etiologies
  - Infection
  - Genetic diseases
  - Metabolic diseases
  - Leukodystrophies
  - Mitochondrial disorders
  - Systemic inflammatory vasculopathies

Treatment

Acute Management

- The mainstay of treatment for acute MS relapses in children is high-dose corticosteroids, which are often administered as intravenous (IV) methylprednisolone (20–30 mg/day) for 3–5 days.[1,11,20]
- Occasionally, this can be followed by a taper of oral prednisone over 2–6 weeks.[1]
- For relapses that do not respond to steroids, therapeutic plasma exchange (typically five single-volume exchanges every other day) or intravenous immune globulin (IVIG) given as 2 g/kg divided over 2–5 days is typically used.[1]
- It is essential to involve physical, occupational, and speech therapy professionals in the acute phase, as they can make recommendations on the frequency and potential duration of inpatient or outpatient therapy.

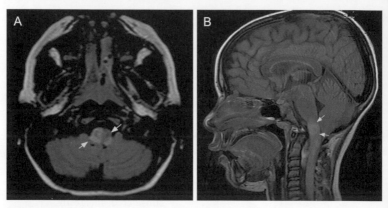

Figure 11.5 Magnetic resonance imaging (MRI) in a pediatric patient with myelin oligodendrocyte glycoprotein (MOG) antibody disease. Axial (A) and sagittal (B) T2/FLAIR images show a brainstem demyelinating lesion (arrows).

- Vitamin D levels should be assessed in all children with ADS or newly diagnosed MS as it is one of the only modifiable risk factors for MS development and relapse.[4]

Chronic Immunomodulatory Treatments

- Fingolimod is the only U.S. Food and Drug Administration (FDA)–approved DMT for use in children at the time of this writing (Table 11.2).
- In general, there are two different approaches to selection of an initial DMT.
  - The "step-up" approach[4,24] involves starting with injectable therapies (interferon beta and glatiramer acetate) and escalating immunotherapy only after patients clinically relapse or show new demyelinating lesions on MRI despite sufficient duration of treatment and validation of compliance by the patient and family.
  - The "step-down" approach[24] involves using the most potent DMTs first despite the potential for some to cause serious adverse events. This approach may be more relevant in children with active disease with significant residual deficits.

Injectable Agents

- Interferon beta agents and glatiramer acetate have the best safety and efficacy data in children. However, approximately 40% of pediatric MS

Table 11.2 Disease-modifying agents used for treatment of pediatric MS. With the exception of fingolimod, all other agents listed are currently used off-label.

	Name	Dose	Side Effects	Monitoring
Injectables	**Interferons** (Rebif, Avonex, Plegridy, Betaseron/Extavia)	**IFNβ-1a**: Avonex: 30 μg IM weekly Rebif: 22 **OR** 44 μg SQ 3x/week **Pegylated IFNβ-1a**: Plegridy: 125 μg SQ every other day **IFNβ-1b**: Betaseron/Extavia: 250 μg SQ every other day	Injection-site reactions, flu-like symptoms, elevated liver enzymes, hematologic abnormalities, thyroid dysfunction	Prior to first dose and every 6 months: CBC, LFT
	Glatiramer acetate (Copaxone)	20 μg SQ daily **OR** 40 μg SQ 3x/ week	Injection-site reactions, post-injection systemic reaction (flushing, chest pain, palpitations, anxiety), skin rash	None
Oral agents	**Fingolimod** (Gilenya)	0.5 mg PO daily	Bradycardia, elevated liver enzymes, macular edema, increased risk for herpes virus infection and PML	EKG at baseline Prior to first dose and every 3 months for the first year: LFT
	Dimethyl fumarate (Tecfidera)	240 mg PO twice daily	Flushing, GI upset, elevated liver enzymes, increased risk for PML.	Prior to first dose and every 6 months: CBC
	Teriflunomide (Aubagio)	7 mg **OR** 14 mg PO daily	GI upset, alopecia, elevated liver enzymes, hypertension, teratogenic	LFT every 6 months.

Table 11.2 (cont.)

	Name	Dose	Side Effects	Monitoring
IV infusions	**Natalizumab** (Tysabri)	300 mg IV every 4 weeks	Infusion reactions, allergic reactions, increased risk for herpes virus infection and PML	Anti-JC virus antibody at baseline and every 6 months MRI every 6–12 months
	Rituximab (Rituxan)	500 mg/m^2 IV × 2 doses 14 days apart **OR** 375 mg/m^2 IV × 4 doses 7 days apart	Infusion reactions, increased risk for herpes virus infection and PML	CBC at baseline and periodically during therapy B-cell levels as clinically indicated
	Alemtuzumab (Lemtrada)	12 mg IV daily × 5 days, then 12 mg IV daily × 3 days one year later	Infusion reactions, autoimmune thyroid disease, ITP, increased risk for herpes virus infection and PML	EKG prior to each treatment course CBC, creatinine, and urinalysis at baseline and monthly until 48 months after last treatment course

Abbreviations: CBC, complete blood count; EKG, electrocardiogram; IM, intramuscular; ITP, immune thrombocytopenic purpura; IV, intravenous; LFT, liver function tests; MRI, magnetic resonance imaging; PML, progressive multifocal leukoencephalopathy; PO, oral (per os); SQ, subcutaneous.

patients treated with these agents will eventually need escalation of therapy.[19,29,32]

- Compliance with self-injectable agents may be an issue in the pediatric population.

- Counseling the family on the medications and providing them with written information to review can allow them to reach an educated decision.

Oral Agents

- In May 2018, fingolimod (Gilenya) became the first FDA-approved immunomodulatory drug for pediatric MS in patients older than age 10.

  - Its approval for this indication was mostly based on results from the PARADIGMS study[3] – the first randomized Phase III clinical trial in pediatric patients (190 children). Side effects were similar to those in adults. with an annual relapse rate reduction of 82% over 2 years.

- Phase III clinical trials for dimethyl fumarate (Tecfidera) and teriflunomide (Aubagio) are currently under way.

Infusion Therapy

- Clinical studies have shown that natalizumab (Tysabri) is effective in children with MS and is associated with significantly reduced MRI activity. In addition, it has a similar side-effect profile in pediatric patients as in adults.[1,9]
- A Phase III clinical trial for alemtuzumab (Lemtrada) is currently ongoing.
- The safety and efficacy of the other infusion therapies remain to be established in children.

Surveillance for Treatment Failure

- Follow-up brain and/or spine MRIs are obtained typically 3–4 months after initiation of DMT to use as baseline to compare to future studies.[27]
- Imaging is then continued at 6 to 12-month intervals.[27] If any of these follow-up studies show new contrast-enhancing or non-enhancing lesions, the possibility of treatment failure should be discussed with the patient and the family.
- It is important to assess treatment compliance and to create a comfortable environment for the patient and family in which to discuss this issue.

  - If noncompliance exists, it is critical to assess barriers to compliance and possibly consider transition to another DMT.
  - If compliance is not an issue, then it is important to discuss transition to another DMT with a potentially more efficacious mechanism.

- Nonradiologic methods for evaluating MS impairment over time include the Multiple Sclerosis Functional Composite (MSFC), which consists of the 9-hole peg test (see Appendix 2), timed 25-foot walk test (see Appendix 3), and Paced Auditory Serial Addition Task (PASAT). The MSFC is typically used in adults, but data on its effectiveness in children are currently lacking.

Symptomatic Management

A diagnosis of MS can have a significant impact on the well-being of both children with MS and their families. The process of receiving a diagnosis may be frustrating and lengthy, and it is essential to provide support and reassurance to the family as well as to address potential misconceptions about the condition. Treatment generally involves a multidisciplinary team of specialists, including neurology, neuropsychology, physical therapy, social work, physical medicine and rehabilitation, nutrition, and school liaison professionals.

Fatigue

- Fatigue is a major symptom in children with MS, which may lead to a poor quality of life.[4,6,11]
- Occupational therapy assessment can be useful to improve any circumstances contributing to the fatigue.
- Pharmacologic agents used in children to treat MS-related fatigue include amantadine, modafinil, fluoxetine, and methylphenidate.[33]

Cognitive Impairment

- Impaired cognition is a common complication of pediatric MS and is important to differentiate from depression and fatigue. It affects school performance and can be mistaken for behavioral issues by teachers.
- Attention, working memory, processing speech, and executive functioning are specific areas of cognitive impairment in children with MS.[24]
- Neuropsychological testing is an important tool to identify a child's relative strengths and weaknesses. It is recommended at baseline and then serially to monitor disease progression.[6,11]
- School liaisons and social workers can help implement recommendations from neuropsychological testing through individualized education plans and 504 plans, in addition to school-based physical and occupational therapy, as well as speech/language pathology services.
- Possible recommendations may include preferential seating, additional time to complete assignments and tests, flexibility in bathroom breaks, and allowing school absences for medical issues.

Mood

- Some children with MS develop anxiety or depression and require consultation and treatment by a pediatric psychiatrist.[33]

- Mood disorders can lead to poor academic performance, oppositional behavior, and social withdrawal in children and adolescents with MS.
- In addition to counseling and pharmacologic treatments, many children and families with MS can greatly benefit from participation in support and educational groups focused on pediatric MS. These activities can help decrease their feelings of isolation and help normalize the condition.

Bladder and Bowel Management

- Urinary dysfunction can be disabling to school-age children. If symptoms do not respond to conservative treatment, evaluation by a urologist and urodynamic testing can be helpful in characterizing the type of urinary dysfunction and guiding therapeutic decision making.[20]
- Constipation can be managed with dietary fiber, bulking agents, stool softeners, promotility agents, enemas, and suppositories.[4]
- As children enter adolescence, it is crucial to foster a trusting relationship with their medical providers so they can speak more freely about issues concerning bowel, bladder, and sexual function.[4]

Pain and Spasticity

- Fortunately, pain does not seem to be as prominent of an issue in children with MS compared to their adult counterparts.[4]
- If pain is reported, a detailed history on the quality and characteristics of the pain can help identify and develop strategies to manage chronic pain.
- Neuropathic pain may respond to medications including gabapentin, tricyclic antidepressants. and serotonin–norepinephrine reuptake inhibitors.[4]
- Pain related to spasticity may respond better to antispasmodic agents, such as baclofen, tizanidine, or dantrolene. Botox injections can be considered for localized areas of spasticity.[34]
- Musculoskeletal pain may be evaluated by physical therapists and physical and rehabilitation specialists, who can identify the need for orthotic devices.

Prognosis

- Disability progression is highly variable in children with MS.[1]
- Some studies suggest that a younger age at diagnosis is associated with slower disease progression in terms of disability. However, a younger age at diagnosis has also been correlated with lower IQ scores.[24]

- There seems to be a higher annualized relapse rate in children with MS compared to adults.[3]
- Approximately 30–40% of children with MS will develop mood disorders, and as many as 75% will have early cognitive impairment.[4]
- Although progression to disability (as measured by the Expanded Disability Status Scale [EDSS]) takes longer in children than in adults, pediatric patients accumulate disability at a younger age compared to adults.[4]

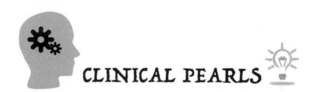

CLINICAL PEARLS

- Diagnosing MS is especially challenging in prepubescent children due to the potential for atypical clinical and radiographic presentations in addition to the broader spectrum of possible differential diagnoses.
- There seems to be a higher annualized relapse rate in children with MS compared to adults.
- The McDonald criteria should be applied with caution in children younger than 12 years, as these criteria have not been validated in this population.
- In children with encephalopathy and multifocal neurologic deficits, ADEM should be suspected.
- Although most children will not have recurring disease after a single demyelinating event, close longitudinal monitoring is warranted in all cases.

References

1. Narula S, Banwell B. Pediatric demyelination. *Continuum (Minneap Minn)*. 2016;22 (3):897–915. doi:10.1212/CON.0000000000000326

2. Ge Y. Multiple sclerosis: the role of MR imaging. *Am J Neuroradiol*. 2006;27(6):1165–76. doi:27/6/1165 [pii]

3. Rostásy K, Bajer-Kornek B. Paediatric multiple sclerosis and other acute demyelinating diseases. *Curr Opin Neurol*. 2018;31(3):244–8. doi:10.1097/ WCO.0000000000000562

4. Wang CX, Greenberg BM. Pediatric multiple sclerosis. *Neurol Clin.* 2018;36:135–149.

5. Polman CH, Reingold SC, Banwell B, et al. Diagnostic criteria for multiple sclerosis: 2010 revisions to the McDonald criteria. *Ann Neurol.* 2011;69(2):292–302. doi:10.1002/ana.22366

6. Cappa R, Theroux L, Brenton JN. Pediatric multiple sclerosis: genes, environment, and a comprehensive therapeutic approach. *Pediatr Neurol.* 2017;75:17–28. doi:10.1016/j.pediatrneurol.2017.07.005

7. Brownlee WJ, Hardy TA, Fazekas F, Miller DH. Diagnosis of multiple sclerosis: progress and challenges. *Lancet.* 2017;389:1336–46. doi:10.1016/S0140-6736(16) 30959-X

8. Milo R, Miller A. Revised diagnostic criteria of multiple sclerosis. *Autoimmun Rev.* 2014;13(4-5):518–24. doi:10.1016/j.autrev.2014.01.012

9. Weber MS, Derfuss T, Metz I, Brück W. Therapeutic advances in neurological disorders. *Ther Adv Neurol Disord.* 2018;11:1–15. doi:10.1177/1756285609104792

10. Balashov K. Imaging of central nervous system demyelinating disorders. *Continuum (Minneap Minn).* 2016;22(5):1613–35. doi:10.1212/ CON.0000000000000373

11. Yamamoto E, Ginsberg M, Rensel M, Moodley M. Pediatric-onset multiple sclerosis: a single center study. *J Child Neurol.* 2018;33(1):98–105. doi:10.1177/ 0883073817739789

12. Tremlett H, Zhao Y, Rieckmann P, Hutchinson M. New perspectives in the natural history of multiple sclerosis. *Neurology.* 2010;74(24):2004–15. doi:10.1212/ WNL.0b013e3181e3973f

13. Thompson AJ, Baranzini SE, Geurts J, et al. Multiple sclerosis. *Lancet Neurol.* 2018;391:1622–36. doi:10.1016/B978-0-7234 3748 2.00015-3

14. Eriksson M, Andersen O, Runmarker B. Long-term follow up of patients with clinically isolated syndromes, relapsing-remitting and secondary progressive multiple sclerosis. *Mult Scler.* 2003;9:260–74.

15. Hollenbach JA, Oksenberg JR. The immunogenetics of multiple sclerosis: a comprehensive review. *J Autoimmun.* 2015;64:13–25. doi:10.1016/j. clinbiochem.2015.06.023.Gut-Liver

16. Okuda DT, Mowry EM, Beheshtian A, et al. Incidental MRI anomalies suggestive of multiple sclerosis. *Neurology.* 2009;72(9):800–5. doi:10.1212/01. wnl.0000335764.14513.1a

17. Olek MJ. Differential diagnosis, clinical features, and prognosis of multiple sclerosis. *Curr Clin Neurol Mult Scler.* 2005:15–53.

18. Gabelic T, Ramasamy DP, Hagemeier J, et al. Prevalence of radiologically isolated syndrome and white matter signal abnormalities in healthy relatives of patients with multiple sclerosis. *Am J Neuroradiol.* 2014;35(1):106–12.

19. Hintzen RQ. Pediatric acquired CNS demyelinating syndromes. *Neurology*. 2016;87: s67–73. doi:10.1212/WNL.0000000000002881

20. Absoud M, Greenberg BM, Lim M, et al. Pediatric transverse myelitis. *Neurology*. 2016;87(9):S46–52. doi:10.1212/WNL.0000000000002820

21. Reich DS, Lucchinetti CF, Calabresi PA. Multiple sclerosis. *N Engl J Med*. 2018;378 (2):169–80. doi:10.1056/NEJMra1401483

22. Marcus JF, Waubant EL. Updates on clinically isolated syndrome and diagnostic criteria for multiple sclerosis. *Neurohospitalist*. 2013;3(2):65–80. doi:10.1177/ 1941874412457183

23. Cross AH, Naismith RT. Established and novel disease-modifying treatments in multiple sclerosis. *J Intern Med*. 2014;275(4):350–63. doi:10.1111/joim.12203

24. Neuteboom R, Wilbur C, Van Pelt D, et al. The spectrum of inflammatory acquired demyelinating syndromes in children. *Semin Pediatr Neurol*. 2017;24(3):189–200. doi:10.1016/j.spen.2017.08.007

25. Baumann M, Grams A, Djurdjevic T, et al. MRI of the first event in pediatric acquired demyelinating syndromes with antibodies to myelin oligodendrocyte glycoprotein. *J Neurol*. 2018;265(4):845–55. doi:10.1007/s00415-018-8781-3

26. Fernandez-Carbonell C, Vargas-Lowy D, Musallam A, et al. Clinical and MRI phenotype of children with MOG antibodies. *Mult Scler J*. 2016;22(2):174–184.

27. Tardieu M, Banwell B, Wolinsky JS, et al. Consensus definitions for pediatric MS and other demyelinating disorders in childhood. *Neurology*. 2016;87(9):S8–11. doi:10.1212/WNL.0000000000002877

28. Sorte DE, Poretti A, Newsome SD, et al. Longitudinally extensive myelopathy in children. *Pediatr Radiol*. 2015;45(2):244–57. doi:10.1007/s00247-014-3225-4

29. Narula S, Banwell B. Pediatric demyelination. *Contin Lifelong Learn Neurol*. 2016;22 (3):897–915. doi:10.1212/CON.0000000000000326

30. Peschl P, Bradl M, Höftberger R, et al. Myelin oligodendrocyte glycoprotein: deciphering a target in inflammatory demyelinating diseases. *Front Immunol*. 2017;8:529. doi:10.3389/fimmu.2017.00529

31. Zhou L, Huang Y, Li H, et al. MOG-antibody associated demyelinating disease of the CNS: a clinical and pathological study in Chinese Han patients. *J Neuroimmunol*. 2017;305:19–28. doi:10.1016/j.jneuroim.2017.01.007

32. Venkateswaran S, Banwell B. Clinical trials in pediatric multiple sclerosis: overcoming the challenges. *Clin Investig (Lond)*. 2013;3:49–56.

33. Yeh EA. Fatigue in childhood multiple sclerosis. *Dev Med Child Neurol*. 2016;58 (3):218. doi:10.1111/dmcn.13055

34. Sarioglu B, Serdaroglu G, Tutuncuoglu S, Ozer EA. The use of botulinum toxin type A treatment in children with spasticity. *Pediatr Neurol*. 2003;29(4):299–301. doi:10.1016/S0887-8994(03)00269-8

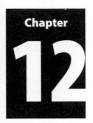

Chapter

12

Useful Websites

Carlos A. Pérez, MD

General Information

- **National Multiple Sclerosis Society** (NMSS; www.nmss.org)

  . NMSS provides information for newly diagnosed individuals and their physicians, treatment options, webcasts, details on current research, and links to local chapters and providers.

- **Multiple Sclerosis Foundation** (MSF; www.msfocus.org)

  . MSF offers programming and support to help patients with MS maintain their independence and make their homes safe. It also provides a variety of other resources, including free booklets on a range of topics that include pregnancy, nutrition, exercise, cognition, and tips for coping with the diagnosis, among others.

Communities, Forums, and Message Boards

- **MSWorld** (www.MSWorld.org)

  . MSWorld is the official message board and chat center for the NMSS. It offers an online MS magazine with stories from patients with MS, book reviews, weblinks, and more. It has dozens of forums and subforums, including a General MS Q&A section.

- **Patients Like Me** (www.patientslikeme.com)

  . This private website allows users to find other patients with MS who share their symptoms, treatments, MS type, and other filterable topics. It also offers a symptom tracker complete with graphs that can be combined with medications.

Newsletters

- **Multiple Sclerosis News Today** (www.multiplesclerosisnewstoday.com)

  . This website presents stories in detail and covers MS-related science
    and research news for patients and their families. It also features a
    variety of forums, MS therapy trackers, and social clips.

Pediatric Multiple Sclerosis

For Children

- **Oscar the MS Monkey** (www.mroscarmonkey.org)

  . This nonprofit organization advocates for and supports children
    diagnosed with MS and their families by raising awareness of pediatric
    MS. Oscar was created by Emily Bolsberg, who was diagnosed with
    MS at the age of 15; she first created him using a pair of orange
    hunting socks. Oscar has become a friend to many children with MS
    since then. He also has a blog and a Facebook page that help children
    connect with other understanding friends.

For Teens

- **Partners Pediatric MS Center** (www.partnersmscenter.org/)

  . The Partners Pediatric MS Center gives teens an opportunity to chat
    with other teens who have MS. There is a monthly online discussion
    group moderated by David Rintell, a psychologist at the Center, which
    takes place on the website MSWorld.org; a special code is required to
    log in.

For the Entire Family

- **National MS Society** (www.nationalMSsociety.org/What-is- MS/Who-
  Gets-MS/Pediatric-MS)

  . This website provides information on pediatric and teen online
    support groups, where children and adolescents can share concerns
    and other information. Its Facebook group also offers a means for
    teens to connect with other teens.

  . **The MS Kids Camp** is a yearly event that is a great opportunity for
    kids who have a parent or guardian with MS to connect with each
    other in a fun and supportive environment.

- **Pediatric MS Online Group for Parents** (www.MSconnection.org)
- **Pediatric Multiple Sclerosis Alliance** (PMSA; http://pediatricms.org)

- The PMSA is dedicated to families of kids, teens, and young adults with MS. It helps families find information, including how and where to connect with others for support.

- **International Pediatric Multiple Sclerosis Study Group** (IPMSSG; http://ipmssg.org/patients/)

    - The IPMSSG is a global network of adult and pediatric neurologists, clinicians, and members of other MS societies, whose mission is to improve the care of children with MS and other demyelinating diseases worldwide. Its website offers information about MS for patients, as well as research, educational events, and other related activities.

Appendices

Carlos A. Pérez, MD

Appendix 1: Expanded Disability Status Scale (EDSS)

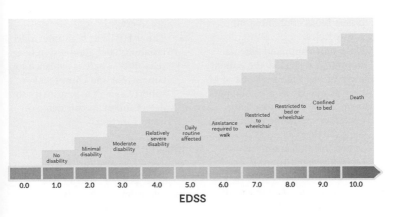

No disability | Minimal disability | Moderate disability | Relatively severe disability | Daily routine affected | Assistance required to walk | Restricted to wheelchair | Restricted to bed or wheelchair | Confined to bed | Death

0.0 1.0 2.0 3.0 4.0 5.0 6.0 7.0 8.0 9.0 10.0

EDSS

References

National Multiple Sclerosis Society. Kurtske Expanded Disability Status Scale. www.nationalmssociety.org/nationalmssociety/media/msnationalfiles/brochures/10-2-3-29-edss_form.pdf

Appendix 2: Nine-Hole Peg Test (9-HPT)

- The 9-HPT is a brief standardized test of upper-extremity function. It tests both the dominant and non-dominant hands twice.

- The patient is seated at a table with a small, shallow container holding nine pegs and a wood or plastic block containing nine empty holes.

- On a start command when a stopwatch is started, the patient picks up the nine pegs one at a time as quickly as possible, puts them in the nine holes, and, once they are in the holes, removes them again as quickly as possible one at a time, replacing them into the shallow container.

- The total time to complete the task is recorded. Two consecutive trials with the dominant hand are immediately followed by two consecutive trials with the nondominant hand.

- The score is an average of the four trials. The two trials for each hand are averaged, converted to the reciprocals of the mean times for each hand, and then the two reciprocals are averaged.

- The 9-HPT has high inter-rater reliability and good test–retest reliability. There is evidence for concurrent and convergent validity as well as sensitivity to detect minor impairments of hand function.

Reference

National Multiple Sclerosis Society. 9-hole peg test (9-HPT). www.nationalmssociety.org/For-Professionals/Researchers/Resources-for-Researchers/Clinical-Study-Measures/9-Hole-Peg-Test-(9-HPT)

Appendix 3: Timed Twenty-Five-Foot Walk Test (T25-FW)

- The T25-FW is a quantitative mobility and leg function performance test based on a timed 25-foot walk.
- The patient is directed to one end of a marked 25-foot course and is instructed to walk 25 feet as quickly and safely as possible.
- The time is calculated from the initiation of the instruction to start and ends when the patient has reached the 25-foot mark.
- The task is immediately administered again by having the patient walk back the same distance.
- Patients may use assistive devices when doing this task.
- Administration time will vary depending on the patient's ability. Total administration time should be approximately 1–5 minutes.

- The score for the T25-FW is the average of the two completed trials.
- Gait speed in general has been demonstrated to be a useful and reliable functional measure of walking ability (and the time to complete the task).
- The T25-FW has high inter-rater and test–retest reliability and shows evidence of good concurrent validity.

Reference

National Multiple Sclerosis Society. Timed 25-foot walk test (T25-FW). www.nationalmssociety.org/For-Professionals/Researchers/Resources-for-Researchers/Clinical-Study-Measures/Timed-25-Foot-Walk-(T25-FW)

Appendix 4: Modified Rio Score Criteria

1. At one year:
   a. **MRI criterion**
      i. 1 point if the patient has had more than five new T2 lesions
   b. **Relapse criterion**
      i. 1 point if the patient experienced one relapse
      ii. 2 points if the patient experienced two or more relapses
2. Score:
   a. ≥2 identifies nonresponders
   b. =1 suggests indeterminate response. Requires reevaluation at 6 months:
      i. Considered a responder if one or more new lesions on repeat magnetic resonance imaging (MRI) and no relapses
      ii. Considered a nonresponder if two or more new lesions or have a relapse
   c. =0 represent responders

References

1. Rio J, Comabella M, Montalban X. Predicting responders to therapies for multiple sclerosis. *Nat Rev Neurol.* 2009;5:553–60.

2. Sormani MP, Rio J, Tintorè M, et al. Scoring treatment response in patients with relapsing multiple sclerosis. *Mult Scler.* 2013;19 (5):605–12.

Index